Parke, Davis & Co.

ORGAN DIRECTED TOXICITIES
OF ANTICANCER DRUGS

DEVELOPMENTS IN ONCOLOGY

W. Davis, C. Maltoni and S. Tanneberger, eds.: The Control of Tumor Growth and its Biological Bases. 0-89838-603-9.
A.P.M. Heintz, C. Th. Griffiths and J.B. Trimbos, eds.: Surgery in Gynecological Oncology. 0-89838-604-7.
M.P. Hacker, E.B. Douple and I. Krakoff, eds.: Platinum Coordination Complexes in Cancer Chemotherapy. 0-89838-619-5.
M.J. van Zwieten. The Rat as Animal Model in Breast Cancer Research: A Histopathological Study of Radiation- and Hormone-Induced Rat Mammary Tumors. 0-89838-624-1.
B. Lowenberg and A. Hogenbeck, eds.: Minimal Residual Disease in Acute Leukemia. 0-89838-630-6.
I. van der Waal and G.B. Snow, eds.: Oral Oncology. 0-89838-631-4.
B.W. Hancock and A.M. Ward, eds.: Immunological Aspects of Cancer. 0-89838-664-0.
K.V. Honn and B.F. Sloane, eds.: Hemostatic Mechanisms and Metastasis. 0-89838-667-5.
K.R. Harrap, W. Davis and A.N. Calvert, eds.: Cancer Chemotherapy and Selective Drug Development. 0-89838-673-X.
V.D. Velde, J.H. Cornelis and P.H. Sugarbaker, eds.: Liver Metastasis. 0-89838-648-5.
D.J. Ruiter, K. Welvaart and S. Ferrone, eds.: Cutaneous Melanoma and Precursor Lesions. 0-89838-689-6.
S.B. Howell, ed.: Intra-Arterial and Intracavitary Cancer Chemotherapy. 0-89838-691-8.
D.L. Kisner and J.F. Smyth, eds.: Interferon Alpha-2: Pre-Clinical and Clinical Evaluation. 0-89838-701-9.
P. Furmanski, J.C. Hager and M.A. Rich, eds.: RNA Tumor Viruses, Oncogenes, Human Cancer and Aids: On the Frontiers of Understanding. 0-89838-703-5.
J.E. Talmadge, I.J. Fidler and R.K. Oldham: Screening for Biological Response Modifiers: Methods and Rationale. 0-89838-712-4.
J.C. Bottino, R.W. Opfell and F.M. Muggia, eds.: Liver Cancer. 0-89838-713-2.
P.K. Pattengale, R.J. Lukes and C.R. Taylor, eds.: Lymphoproliferative Diseases: Pathogenesis, Diagnosis, Therapy. 0-89838-725-6.
F. Cavalli, G. Bonadonna and M. Rozencweig, eds.: Malignant Lymphomas and Hodgkin's Disease. 0-89838-727-2.
L. Baker, F. Valeriote and V. Ratanatharathorn, eds.: Biology and Therapy of Acute Leukemia. 0-89838-728-0.
J. Russo, ed.: Immunocytochemistry in Tumor Diagnosis. 0-89838-737-X.
R.L. Ceriani, ed.: Monoclonal Antibodies and Breast Cancer. 0-89838-739-6.
D.E. Peterson, G.E. Elias and S.T. Sonis, eds.: Head and Neck Management of the Cancer Patient. 0-89838-747-7.
D.M. Green: Diagnosis and Management of Malignant Solid Tumors in Infants and Children. 0-89838-750-7.
K.A. Foon and A.C. Morgan, Jr., eds.: Monoclonal Antibody Therapy of Human Cancer. 0-89838-754-X.
J.G. McVie, et al, eds.: Clinical and Experimental Pathology of Lung Cancer. 0-89838-764-7.
K.V. Honn, W.E. Powers and B.F. Sloane, eds.: Mechanisms of Cancer Metastasis. 0-89838-765-5.
K. Lapis, L.A. Liotta and A.S. Rabson, eds.: Biochemistry and Molecular Genetics of Cancer Metastasis. 0-89838-785-X.
A.J. Mastromarino, ed.: Biology and Treatment of Colorectal Cancer Metastasis. 0-89838-786-8.
M.A. Rich, J.C. Hager and J. Taylor-Papadimitriou, eds.: Breast Cancer: Origins, Detection, and Treatment. 0-89838-792-2.
D.G. Poplack, L. Massimo and P. Cornaglia-Ferraris, eds.: The Role of Pharmacology in Pediatric Oncology. 0-89838-795-7.
A. Hagenbeek and B. Lowenberg, eds.: Minimal Residual Disease in Acute Leukemia 1986. 0-89838-799-X.
F.M. Muggia and M. Rozencweig, eds.: Clinical Evaluations of Anti-Tumor Therapy. 0-89838-803-1.
F.A. Valeriote and L.H. Baker, eds.: Biochemical Modulation of Anticancer Agents: Experimental and Clinical Approaches. 0-89838-827-9.
B.A. Stoll, ed.: Pointers to Cancer Prognosis. 0-89838-841-4.
K.H. Hollman and J.M. Verley, eds.: New Frontiers in Mammary Pathology 1986. 0-89838-852-X.
D.J. Ruiter, G.J. Fleuren and S.O. Warneer, eds.: Application of Monoclonal Antibodies in Tumor Pathology. 0-89838-853-8.
A.H.G. Paterson and A.W. Lees, eds.: Fundamental Problems in Breast Cancer. 0-89838-863-5.

ORGAN DIRECTED TOXICITIES OF ANTICANCER DRUGS

Proceedings of the First International Symposium on the Organ Directed Toxicities of Anticancer Drugs Burlington, Vermont, USA-June 4–6, 1987

edited by

Miles P. Hacker
Vermont Regional Cancer Center
Burlington, Vermont

John S. Lazo
Yale University School of Medicine
New Haven, Connecticut

Thomas R. Tritton
Vermont Regional Cancer Center
Burlington, Vermont

Martinus Nijhoff Publishing
a member of the Kluwer Academic Publishers Group
Boston/Dordrecht/Lancaster

Distributors for North America:
Kluwer Academic Publishers
101 Philip Drive
Assinippi Park
Norwell, Massachusetts 02061 USA

Distributors for the UK and Ireland:
Kluwer Academic Publishers
MTP Press Limited
Falcon House, Queen Square
Lancaster LA1 1RN, UNITED KINGDOM

Distributors for all other countries:
Kluwer Academic Publishers Group
Distribution Centre
Post Office Box 322
3300 AH Dordrecht, THE NETHERLANDS

Library of Congress Cataloging-in-Publication Data

International Symposium on the Organ Directed Toxicities of Anticancer
Drugs (1st : 1987 : Burlington, Vt.)
  Organ directed toxicities of anticancer drugs : proceedings of the
First International Symposium on the Organ Directed Toxicities of
Anticancer Drugs, convened in Burlington, Vermont by the Vermont
Regional Cancer Center, June 4-6, 1987 / edited by Miles P. Hacker,
John S. Lazo, Thomas R. Tritton.
     p. cm. — (Developments in oncology)
  Includes bibliographies and indexes.
  ISBN 0-89838-356-0
  1. Cancer—Chemotherapy—Congresses.   2. Antineoplastic agents—
Side effects—Congresses.   3. Heart—Effect of drugs on—
Congresses. 4. Lungs—Effect of drugs on—Congresses.   5. Kidneys—
Effect of drugs on—Congresses. I. Hacker, Miles P. II. Lazo,
John S. III. Tritton, Thomas R. IV. Vermont Regional Cancer
Center. V. Title. VI. Series.
  [DNLM: 1. Antineoplastic Agents—adverse effects—congresses.
2. Heart—drug effects—congresses. 3. Kidney—drug effects—
congresses. W1 DE998N / QV 269 I605 1987o]
RC271.C51556 1988
616.99 '4061—dc19
DNLM/DLC   87-31391
for Library of Congress   CIP

Printed in the United States of America

SYMPOSIUM COMMITTEES

SPONSORS

The symposium was supported in part by a Grant,
#1 R13 CA43865-01, from the National Cancer Institute.

CONTRIBUTORS

MARLENE ABSHER, Department of Medicine, College of Medicine, University of Vermont, Burlington, Vermont   05405

ROBERT S. BENJAMIN, University of Texas System, M.D. Anderson Hospital and Tumor Institute at Houston, Houston, Texas   77030

RONALD R. BLUM, Kaplan Cancer Center, New York University, 530 East Avenue, New York, New York   10016

RICHARD F. BORCH, Department of Pharmacology and Cancer Center, University of Rochester, Rochester, New York   14642

C. HUMBERTO CARRASCO, University of Texas System, M.D. Anderson Hospital and Tumor Institute at Houston, Houston, Texas   77030

JOHN D. CATRAVAS, Department of Pharmacology and Toxicology, Medical College of Georgia, Augusta, Georgia   30912

SANT P. CHAWLA, University of Texas System, M.D. Anderson Hospital and Tumor Institute at Houston, Houston, Texas   77030

DEBRA COCKAYNE, Department of Biochemistry, College of Medicine, University of Vermont, Burlington, Vermont   05405

KENNETH R. CUTRONEO, Department of Biochemistry, College of Medicine, University of Vermont, Burlington, Vermont   05405

PETER C. DEDON, Department of Pharmacology and Cancer Center, University of Rochester, Rochester, New York   14642

JAMES H. DOROSHOW, Department of Medical Oncology and Therapeutics Research, City of Hope Cancer Research Center, Duarte, California   91010

NEIL DUBIN, Kaplan Cancer Center, Department of Medicine, New York University, 530 East Avenue, New York, New York   10016

MICHAEL S. EWER, University of Texas System, M.D. Anderson Hospital and Tumor Institute at Houston, Houston, Texas   77030

FREDERICK FEIT, Department of Cardiology, New York University, 530 East Avenue, New York, New York   10016

VICTOR J. FERRANS, Ultrastructure Section, Pathology Branch, National Heart, Lung and Blood Institute, National Institutes of Health, Bethesada, Maryland   20892

RONALD GORDON, Department of Pathology, Mount Sinai School of Medicine, New York, New York   10029

MICHAEL D. GREEN, Kaplan Cancer Center, Department of Medicine, New York University, 530 East Avenue, New York, New York   10016

ARTHUR P. GROLLMAN, Department of Pharmacological Sciences, State University of New York at Stony Brook, Stony Brook, New York   11794

MILES P. HACKER, Department of Pharmacology and Vermont Regional Cancer Center, University of Vermont, Burlington, Vermont   05401

ROBERT L. HAMLIN, College of Veterinary Medicine, Ohio State University, Columbus, Ohio 43210

EUGENE H. HERMAN, Division of Drug Biology, Food and Drug Administration, Washington, DC   20204

GABRIEL N. HORTOBAGYI, University of Texas System, M.D. Anderson Hospital and Tumor Institute at Houston, Houston, Texas   77030

ANN JACQUOTTE, Kaplan Cancer Center, Department of Medicine, New York University, 530 East Avenue, New York, New York   10016

JASON KELLEY, Department of Medicine, College of Medicine, University of Vermont, Burlington, Vermont   05405

ELIZABETH J. KOVACS, Department of Anatomy, Loyola University Medical Center, Maywood, Illinois   60153

IRWIN H. KRAKOFF, University of Texas System Cancer Center, M.D. Anderson Hospital and Tumor Institute, 1515 Holcombe Boulevard, Houston, Texas   77030

ELISSA KRAMER, Department of Nuclear Medicine, New York University, 530 East Avenue, New York, New York   10016

JOHN S. LAZO, Department of Pharmacology, Yale University School of Medicine, 333 Cedar Street, New Haven, Connecticut   06510

SEWA S. LEGHA, University of Texas System, M.D. Anderson Hospital and Tumor Institute at Houston, Houston, Texas   77030

CHARLES L. LITTERST, Laboratory of Experimental Therapeutics and Metabolism, National Cancer Institute, National Institutes of Health, Bethesda, Maryland   20892

CAROLE LONDON, Kaplan Cancer Center, New York University, 530 East Avenue, New York, New York   10016

BRUCE MACKAY, University of Texas System, M.D. Anderson Hospital and Tumor Institute at Houston, Houston, Texas   77030

MARLEEN MEYERS, Kaplan Cancer Center, New York University, 530 East Avenue, New York, New York   10016

JOHN E. MIGNANO, Department of Pharmacology, Yale University School of Medicine, 333 Cedar Street, New Haven, Connecticut   06510

THOMAS J. MONTINE, Department of Pharmacology and Cancer Center, University of Rochester, Rochester, New York   14642

FRANCO M. MUGGIA, Kaplan Cancer Center, New York University, 530 East Avenue, New York, New York   10016

CHARLES E. MYERS, Clinical Pharmacology Branch, National Cancer Institute, National Institutes of Health, Bethesda, Maryland   20892

ROBERT F. OZOLS, Division of Cancer Treatment, National Cancer Institute, National Institutes of Health, Bethesda, Maryland   20892

MIRIAM C. POIRIER, Division of Cancer Etiology, National Cancer Institute, National Institutes of Health, Bethesda, Maryland   20892

EDDIE REED, Division of Cancer Treatment, National Cancer Institute, National Institutes of Health, Bethesda, Maryland   20892

MARIANO REY, Department of Radiology, New York University, 530 East Avenue, New York, New York   10016

ROBERT SAFIRSTEIN, Department of Medicine, Mount Sinai School of Medicine, New York, New York   10029

JOSEPH SANGER, Department of Radiology, New York University, 530 East Avenue, New York, New York   10016

SAID M. SEBTI, Department of Pharmacology, Yale University School of Medicine, 333 Cedar Street, New Haven, Connecticut   06510

JAMES L. SPEYER, Kaplan Cancer Center, Department of Medicine, New York University, 530 East Avenue, New York, New York   10016

PETER STECY, Department of Cardiology, New York University, 530 East Avenue, New York, New York   10016

KENNETH M. STERLING, JR., Department of Pediatrics and Biochemistry, Mount Sinai School of Medicine, New York, New York   10029

SUSAN TAUBES, Kaplan Cancer Center, New York University, 530 East Avenue, New York, New York   10016

THOMAS R. TRITTON, Department of Pharmacology and Vermont Regional Cancer Center, University of Vermont, Burlington, Vermont   05401

A. FRANCINE TRYKA, Department of Pathology, Arkansas Children's Hospital and University of Arkansas for Medical Sciences, Little Rock, Arkansas   72207

SIDNEY WALLACE, University of Texas System, M.D. Anderson Hospital and Tumor Institute at Houston, Houston, Texas   77030

CYNTHIA WARD, Kaplan Cancer Center, Department of Medicine, New York University, 530 East Avenue, New York, New York   10016

JAMES C. WERNZ, Kaplan Cancer Center, New York University, 530 East Avenue, New York, New York   10016

ROBERT C. YOUNG, Division of Cancer Treatment, National Cancer Institute, National Institutes of Health, Bethesda, Maryland   20892

ARTHUR Z. ZELENT, Departments of Medicine and Biochemistry, Mount Sinai School of Medicine, New York, New York   10029

PREFACE

The addition of chemotherapy as an effective means to treat cancer has had a major impact on selected human malignancies. Due to a general inability to differentiate between normal and neoplastic cells, little selectivity exists in currently used oncolytic drugs. Consequently, significant toxicity to the patient is expected when systemic cancer chemotherapy is chosen as an appropriate therapeutic intervention. Much of this toxicity, such as damage to the bone marrow, gastrointestinal tract, or hair follicles, is predictable based upon the fact that anticancer drugs kill actively dividing cells. These types of toxicities, while serious, are usually manageable and reversible and are, therefore, not often considered to be dose limiting.

Unfortunately, several of the most important anticancer drugs also damage tissues in which the growth fraction is relatively small. Such toxicities can not be predicted based on the chemical structure of the drugs, are often not detected in preclinical studies, and are encountered frequently for the first time in clinical studies. Further, unlike most of the proliferative-dependent toxicities, the unpredicted toxicities are usually irreversible or only partially reversible upon cessation of drug administration. Because of this, the unpredicted toxicities are referred to as dose limiting. They represent a significant barrier to the ultimate efficacy of several of our most important anticancer drugs.

Significant research effort has been directed toward developing a better understanding of the mechanisms of such dose limiting toxicities. For some drugs, this knowledge has resulted in clinically effective ways to diminish specific toxicities. In others, no such inroads have been made. In spite of the clinical importance and the extent of research expended to date, no symposium had been convened at which investigators from various disciplines could meet to discuss research observations and concepts. Recognizing this, the First International Symposium on Organ Directed Toxicities of Anticancer Drugs was convened by the Vermont Regional Cancer Center in Burlington, Vermont on June 4-6, 1987. In order to provide focus to this meeting, the organizers chose to concentrate on the heart, lung and kidney as the sites of dose limiting toxicities.

This volume includes the manuscripts of the invited speakers from each of the three sessions. Mechanisms of toxicities and approaches to diminishing toxicities of each of the organs mentioned above are described. The speakers were requested to review recent developments and to highlight new areas of focus and promise. The abstracts of the scientific posters that were presented at the symposium are also included.

x

The editors wish to thank the contributors for their timely presentations and manuscript preparation. Obviously, this symposium would not have been possible were it not for financial support provided by several sources as acknowledged elsewhere in this volume. The conveners gratefully appreciate this support. Special thanks are also reserved for Joan MacKenzie and Maureen Hanagan who, with support of their respective staffs, provided the local arrangements and general organization necessary for the success of the Symposium.

Miles P. Hacker, John S. Lazo and Thomas R. Tritton

TABLE OF CONTENTS

KEYNOTE ADDRESS

SECTION I: ANTHRACYCLINE INDUCED CARDIOTOXICITY

SECTION II: BLEOMYCIN INDUCED PULMONARY TOXICITY

xii

SECTION III: PLATINUM INDUCED NEPHROTOXICITY

SECTION IV: POSTER PRESENTATIONS

KEYNOTE ADDRESS

I.H. Krakoff

The Irrelevant Toxicities
of Anticancer Drugs
I.H. Krakoff

The origins of cancer chemotherapy are in toxicology. During World War II a unit of the chemical warfare service stationed at the Edgewood Arsenal in Maryland studied poison gases with particular emphasis on the mustards. The unit was headed by Dr. Cornelius P. Rhoads, on leave from his position as Scientific Director of Memorial Hospital. One must assume that in studying the antiproliferative effect of the mustards, Rhoads and his colleagues were, from the beginning, keenly aware of the potential for these compounds as anticancer agents. The animal studies conducted at the Edgewood Arsenal provided a background on which those investigators were able to build, with the major military disaster at Bari, Italy, providing an opportunity to study the toxic effects of nitrogen mustard in a large number of human subjects. During the same period of time a few patients with lymphoma were treated at New Haven with nitrogen mustard and enjoyed dramatic, although brief, remission in their disease. By the end of the war it was clear that a potent agent with significant potential for use as an anticancer drug had been developed.

Toxicity is one of the major problems in the development and use of anticancer compounds.

A more accurate term might be selectivity; since toxicity to tumor cells is the aim of cancer chemotherapy our search is not for non-toxic compounds but rather for compounds which will selectively damage tumor cells without damaging normal mammalian cells. That goal has been achieved in antibacterial chemotherapy. The demonstration of antibacterial properties of sulfanilamide in the 1930's was based on the requirement of certain bacteria for para-aminobenzoic acid. Adequate concentrations of sulfanilamide deprived bacteria of PABA. Human cells, not requiring exogenous PABA, were not damaged by sulfanilamide. This exploitable biochemical difference between bacterial cells and mammalian cells does not have a parallel in a difference between normal human cells and human tumor cells. It is this lack of selectivity, or at least the failure to demonstrate the difference to date, that has made it so difficult to develop non-toxic antitumor drugs. In 1941, William Woglom stated "to think of a systemic treatment for cancer would be almost as difficult as to dissolve the left ear and leave the right ear intact." In 1987, although recognizing the inherent logic of that statement, it is clear that exploitation of quantitative differences between tumor and normal cells has provided some tools with which significant antitumor effects can be obtained with acceptable toxicity to the human host.

Most anticancer drugs, as part of their antiproliferative effect, are regularly toxic to those organ systems which are characterized by active proliferation. These include the bone marrow, the gastrointestinal epithelium, hair follicles, germinal epithelium and lymphoid tissues. Less regular effects are those which occur in organs which are not rapidly growing and in general, through mechanisms other than a direct antiproliferative effect. It is these which appear to be unrelated to antitumor activity which have been called "irrelevant" to the major cytotoxic action of anticancer drugs. Clinically, we are accustomed to myelosuppression as the most common limiting toxicity and are able to use anticancer drugs to the point of marked myelosuppression. The development of effective antibiotic therapy, thrombocyte replacement and autologous bone marrow transplantation have helped to cope with myelosuppression. However, as bone marrow toxicity has become less prominent as a limiting factor, toxicity to other organ systems, some of which are the topics of this symposium, have emerged as major problems. It is assumed, although not yet definitively proven, that elimination of the cardiotoxicity of doxorubicin, the pulmonary toxicity of bleomycin and the nephrotoxicity of cisplatin would make those agents therapeutically more effective. Many of the papers in this symposium will deal with attempts to modify those "irrelevant" toxicities.

In developing new drugs our model animal systems predict very well for toxicity to rapidly proliferating organs. We can predict bone marrow and gastrointestinal toxicity quite well. Animal systems do much less well in predicting for liver and kidney toxicity. It is for that reason that the phase I clinical study must be conducted extremely carefully, looking for, not only those organ toxicities anticipated from the preclinical studies, but also employing broad clinical, biochemical and hematologic screens. Even so, some toxic effects are delayed in onset or may depend on cumulative dose. The cardiotoxicity of doxorubicin was not anticipated from preclinical studies and was not observed in classical phase I studies. Only in phase II trials in which cumulative doses reached 500 to 600 mg/m^2, did cardiac toxicity become apparent, and then it was necessary to go back to animal systems to develop suitable models to study. We assume until proven otherwise that compounds which may exhibit antitumor activity will also be teratogenic, even though that may not be apparent from preclinical studies. Even after the sedative, thalidomide, was observed to be teratogenic in humans, it was extremely difficult to develop an animal model.

The classic phase I study of a new potential anticancer agent is initiated at a regular fraction of the lethal dose in mice. It is the practice in that initial clinical study to escalate the dose gradually in an attempt to determine the maximum tolerated dose (MTD). Subsequent therapeutic trials will be conducted at a dose which is close to the MTD. It has been demonstrated repeatedly in animal systems that virtually every useful antitumor agent has a very steep dose response relationship and it is concluded therefore that the best chance for therapeutic activity is at the highest dose which can be administered. Recent clinical studies lend credence to the view that dose intensity is an important factor in clinical responsiveness.

There are species differences which may cause difficulty in extrapolation from animal to man and there are, as well, differences between individual humans which may cause significant variability

in tolerated dose from patient to patient. Variability
in gastrointestinal absorption may markedly influence
the biologic activity of a drug and until it is
demonstrated that absorption is constant from
patient to patient, it is wise to assume that
it is not. Many secondary factors can influence
drug toxicity. Since doxorubicin is largely excreted
in the bile, liver disease can markedly enhance
the acute toxicity of that drug. X-ray therapy
delivered to the mediastinum can increase the
potential for cardiac toxicity of that drug.
Methotrexate is rapidly excreted through the kidney.
Renal disease which impedes the urinary excretion
of methotrexate can markedly enhance its toxicity.
Allopurinol inhibits xanthine oxidase, the enzyme
responsible for the oxidation of hypoxanthine
and xanthine to uric acid; that same enzyme is
responsible for the oxidative degradation of
6-mercaptopurine to an inert end-product, 6-thiouric
acid. Therefore, patients who receive allopurinol,
a xanthine oxidase inhibitor, for the treatment
of gout or for the prevention of secondary hyper-
uricemia must be given 6-mercaptopurine in reduced
dose to avoid serious toxicity. It was not until
several patients, presumably cured of metastatic
testicular cancer were given oxygen during exploratory
surgery and in the immediate postoperative period,
that it was recognized that oxygen can markedly
enhance the potential for pulmonary toxicity of
bleomycin. It is clear that our evaluation of
drug toxicity does not end with the phase I study,
but extends far into the period of therapeutic
evaluation and clinical use.

It would seem to be a simple feat to eliminate
the organ directed toxicities which are irrelevant

to the antitumor effect of drugs and yet to date that has been very difficult to accomplish. The pulmonary toxicity of bleomycin, the cardiotoxicity of doxorubicin and the neurotoxicity of vincristine continue to require a cap on cumulative dose. Hemorrhagic cystitis, although not a serious problem at conventional doses, becomes a major concern with the administration of cyclophosphamide in the large doses necessary for marrow ablation and bone marrow transplantation. In spite of our therapeutic advances, nephrotoxicity, ototoxicity, peripheral neuropathy and emesis limit the therapeutic use of cisplatin.

There are several ways in which this problem might be addressed. The effort to develop totally new anticancer drugs continues. It is possible that entirely new structures will produce useful therapeutic effects without toxicity; however, it is equally possible that promising new therapeutic agents may exhibit toxicities that we have not yet experienced. Efforts continue to develop analogs of existing drugs which may be more effective and less toxic than those presently in use and to develop specific methods for blocking specific organ toxicities. Several analogs of doxorubicin now in clinical trial are thought to be quantitatively less prone to produce cardiac toxicity and a morph-olino-cyano derivative of doxorubicin, not yet in clinical trial, appears to be approximately 1000 times as potent as doxorubicin without a parallel increase in cardiac toxicity. Several analogs of bleomycin have been studied clinically but without evidence to date that they are free of pulmonary toxicity. A newer analog, liblomycin, appears in animal studies to be considerably superior to bleomycin in that respect; it has recently entered clinical trial in Japan. Two derivatives of cisplatin presently in clinical trial appear to be less nephrotoxic than cisplatin. A group of diaminocyclohexane derivatives of cisplatin appear to be devoid of nephrotoxicity and to offer considerable therapeutic advantage. Those compounds will enter clinical trial in the near future.

Changes in dose schedule may be useful. The cardiotoxicity of doxorubicin, known to be related to cumulative dose, can be modified by schedules which avoid the high peak levels achieved by intermittent bolus administration. Continuous infusion or intermittent lower dose administration appear to achieve therapeutically equal results with a decreased risk of cardiac toxicity. Specific inhibition of organ site toxicity has been effective in specific circumstances. The hemorrhagic cystitis produced by cyclophosphamide and isophosphamide appears to be due to the production of acrolein as one of the degradation products; in Europe, the use of 2-mercaptoethanesulfonate (Mesna) appears to have markedly diminished that problem. Mesna has recently entered clinical trial in the United States. A derivative of cyclophosphamide in which a dithiol moiety is incorporated into the molecule (AZ7557) appears in animal studies not to cause bladder toxicity and to be therapeutically at least as active as the parent compound.

Current efforts at the systemic treatment of cancer are aimed at the destruction of tumor cells. There has been considerable progress toward that end although antiproliferative activity toward tumor cells appears to be intimately associated with antiproliferative activity toward non-tumor cells. The occurrence of other biologic activity has been more difficult to forecast, although it is probably inevitable. As we learn more of the nature of these irrelevant toxicities it seems increasingly likely that they might be eliminated through specific design of analogs and through specific inhibition of their activity on target organs. Until cancer therapies are devised which may be far more specific in their actions against tumor cells, it appears likely that drug toxicity will continue to be a problem.

SECTION I

ANTHRACYCLINE INDUCED CARDIOTOXICITY

Chaired by T.R. Tritton

Overview
T.R. Tritton

When one thinks of anthracyclines, one reflexively associates these drugs with cardiotoxicity. It may in fact be the case that drug resistance or even simple myelosuppression are the problems that most often limit successful therapy with anthracyclines, but nonetheless a great deal of effort in many laboratories around the world has been invested in understanding the mechanism(s) and consequences of cardiac-directed organ toxicity. The five papers in this section approach the problem from several perspectives, including both basic and applied science. Taken together, they provide a broad view of the underlying mechanisms and clinical ramifications associated with cardiotoxicity.

Myers considers the role of iron in anthracycline action. He provides a fascinating historical reflection on iron chelation and its commercial applications, and succinctly summarizes the growing literature on adriamycin/iron chemistry. This chemistry then presages a biochemical foundation for the hypothesis that iron chelation or free radical scavenging could protect against anthracycline cardiotoxicity. Dr. Myers also discusses his own and other laboratories' results suggesting that the various biological actions of the anthracyclines (intercalation, topoisomerase interaction, cytotoxicity, mutagenesis, cardiotoxicity etc.) may be separated by appropriate structural modification. This is good news indeed for chemist and clinician alike, since it provides a powerful impetus to continue to search for new anthracyclines which retain oncolytic activity but which lack the notorious cardiotoxicity.

Doroshow takes as a point of departure the idea that cardiac mitochondria are an important intracellular site for anthracycline cardiotoxicity, and then discusses studies using isolated mitochondria as a model system. Complex I is the principal site of mitochondrial inhibition by adriamycin and the City of Hope group has provided an elegant insight into the detailed biochemistry of this system. In addition, however, NADPH cytochrome P450 dehydrogenase in the sarcoplasmic reticulum and xanthine oxidase in the cytosol are also targets for the drug. Thus there may be several levels of attack open to the anthracyclines in damaging heart muscle, which makes the design of selective ameliorators more difficult. As in Myers' work, Doroshow also provides evidence that membrane or protein bound iron acts as a catalyst for oxyradical formation which is presumed to be a candidate for the active toxic species in cardiac damage.

The remaining three papers in this section describe attempts to lessen or manage the cardiotoxicity of the anthracyclines. Benjamin summarizes the results of an extensive clinical study (>250 patients) where cardiac biopsy and ejection fraction measurements are used to assess toxicity and predict congestive heart failure. The most successful approach to reducing toxicity is a 96 hour continuous infusion of adriamycin. Epirubicin, an anthracycline with a lower intrinsic cardiotoxic potential, was also less toxic by infusion, but a bolus administration of epirubicin was more cardiotoxic than a continuous infusion of adriamycin. This infusion procedure thus defines a new standard against which future attempts to ameliorate cardiotoxicity must be measured.

Ferrans' paper describes the experimental rationale for using ICRF-187 to protect against cardiotoxicity. Unlike previous attempts to block heart damage by free radical scavengers (e.g., vitamin E, N-acetylcysteamine, ubiquinone) ICRF-187 is thought to act by chelation of iron. Removal of iron then prevents metal ion interaction with adriamycin, a step which is presumed necessary for drug mediated formation of free radicals. The active ICRF-187 compound does indeed provide a high degree of protection against otherwise lethal doses of daunorubicin in hamsters, dogs, mice, rats, rabbits and miniature swine. In fact, pretreatment of beagles with ICRF-187 allows subsequent dose escalation of adriamycin up to four-fold higher levels than would normally be considered safe. Indications so far also suggest that ICRF-187 does not by itself cause notable toxicity nor does it reduce the anticancer efficacy of the anthracycline.

The work by Speyer et al. uses the principles developed by Ferrans and his collaborators to design a clinical trial of ICRF-187 in patients with metastatic breast cancer receiving adriamycin as part of their treatment regimen. The results, although preliminary, are encouraging. It appears that cardiotoxic protection has occurred and, most importantly, without lowering the response rate to the drug combination. This represents the first time that an idea originating in the laboratory on anthracycline cardiotoxicity has been taken to the clinic and not been disappointing. The results also raise an interesting dilemma. If iron chelation is the mechanism for cardioprotection, and no antitumor activity is lost to ICRF-187, this may suggest a lessor role for iron in the antitumor mechanism than previously suspected by some workers. It is also possible that pharmacokinetic or distribution differences could account for the results, but whatever the explation, this work raises intriguing possibilities for future investigations.

Role of Iron in
Anthracycline Action
C.E. Myers

INTRODUCTION

While considerable interest has focused on anthracycline free radical formation as a mechanism of toxicity and, more recently, tumor cell kill, it is only relatively recently that attention has focused on the role of iron chemistry in this process. Interest in this problem is bound to increase as a result of recent clinical and preclinical studies which demonstrate that ICRF-187, an EDTA derivative, effectively prevents doxorubicin-induced cardiac toxicity. During its initial phase 1 clinical trial, ICRF-187 was shown to increase urinary iron clearance by more than an order of magnitude. While direct evidence has not been presented which links iron chelation with the ability of this agent to prevent cardiac toxicity, this would have to be considered the leading hypothesis. Prior to these studies, it had been shown that the presence of iron could play and important role in doxorubicin-induced lipid peroxidation.

There has been some controversy as to how iron might participate in doxorubicin-induced free radical injury. One school of thought favored a reaction of free iron with drug and reactive oxygen species. In this hypothesis, the role of iron was viewed as not unique to the anthracyclines, but rather consistent with the known role of iron in general radical chemistry. The other school of thought has postulated that doxorubicin and other anthracyclines formed iron complexes with unusual properties and that the chemistry of these drug-iron complexes was an important determinant of drug action. Over the past several years, our understanding of the properties of the drug-iron complexes has grown rapidly and this chapter will be devoted to a discussion of these results and their implications.

HISTORICAL EVIDENCE

Both doxorubicin and daunomycin are hydroxyquinones and it is important to point out that iron chelation by hydroxyquinones is a general and well established property of this chemical class. This property forms the basis for the mordent method of dying cloth, in which iron or other transition metal ions bind to both cloth and hydroxyquinone dyes, effectively linking the two together. This process was extensively used by both the ancient Egyptians and Romans. Part of the attractiveness of this process is that the dye was often very stable and not removed by repeated washing. At present, this approach is still widely used by those who work with natural dyes. In addition, this process has found wide use at the hands of histochemists as a means to stain specific tissue consitiuents. It should not, therefore, be a surprise that anthracyclines are effectivve chelators of iron and other transition metal ions. Indeed, this property of the anthracyclines was established quite early (1).

TECHNICAL DIFFICULTIES WORKING WITH IRON

Ferric ion presents the investigator with several difficult problems. One of the most serious is that Fe(III) rapidly polymerizes at physiologic pH to form a ferric hydroxide polymer (rust in the common veracular) which are not accessible to metal chaltors (2). As a result, if Fe(III) is mixed with a chelator at physiologic pH, much of the iron is lost to the polymer and the result is a poor yield of the complex. There are two techniques which can be used to overcome this problem. First, the chelator and metal iron can be mixed at an acid pH and then slowly brought up to pH 7.0. The second approach is prepare a complex between iron and a weaker chelator which can then act as a donor to stronger chelator. Two commonly used donor ligands are nitriloacetic acid and acetohlydroxamic acid. We have used either method depending upon the needs of the needs of the experimental protocol (3, 4). It should be pointed out that *in vivo* most iron is in a chelated state, bound to proteins and amino acids.

One of the difficulties in working with doxorubicin is that it binds to glassware, plastic, many proteins, lab equipment, clothing and ski. The doxorubicin-iron complex is even a greater problem and we have found it necessary to wash glassware with 1N HCL and EDTA.

An additional problem is that the doxorubicin-iron complex is quite photoreactive. For example, in studies designed to determine whether the doxorubicin-iron complex cleaved DNA, we found it necessary to work with the overhead fluorescent lights off in order to control light induced DNA cleavage by the drug-metal complex (5).

Finally, the doxorubicin-iron complex is not stable, but degrades over a peroid of hours. Therefore, it is best to make it up fresh prior to each use.

STRUCTURE OF THE DRUG-IRON COMPLEXES

Fe(III) has six d orbitals available for chelation. Monodenate ligands bind to a single d orbital, while bidentate or tridentate ligands can bind to two or three orbitals. For Fe(III), there is a maximum binding capacity of six monodentate, three bidentate and two tridentate ligands. Fe(III) binds a maximum of three doxorubicin and thus the drug is a bidentate ligand (3). This is consistent with the fact that hydroxyquinones usually bind Fe(III) to the carbonyl and -OH. Interaction at this site has been documented laser raman spectroscopy. In addition, terbium(III) which has similar binding requirements to Fe(III), has been shown by NMR to bind at this site.

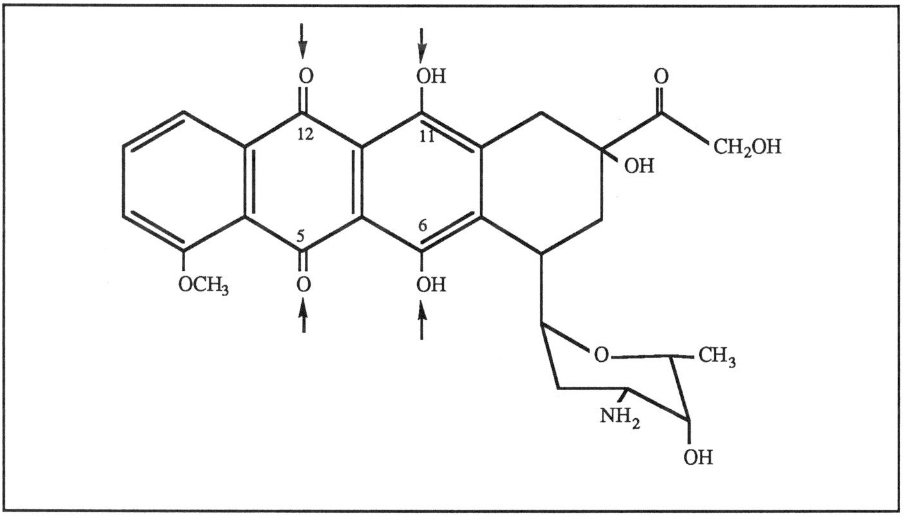

Figure 1. Doxorubicin with chelation sites marked

Based upon the published X-ray crystal structures for the drug, we pointed out that the O-O distances at C5-C6 and C11-C12 were not identical (6). This was confirmed by the different NMR resonances for the protons at C6 and C12. We pointed out that the O-O distance at C11-C12 looked to be a much better fit with Fe(III) than did that at C5-C6. While a preference for C11-C12 has been shown for terbium (III), specific proof of this contention for Fe(III) is lacking. There are other potential iron binding sites on the ketol side chain and at the sugan amino group. Direct evidence for iron binding at these sites has not been presented. At present, X-ray crystallography of the drug-iron complex has not been done.

The published binding constants for the association of the first, second and third doxorubicin are 10^{18}, 10^{11} and $10^{4.4}$ (7). These results indicate that the third doxorubicin is weakly bound and would be easily displaced by a number of other ligands. It is interesting to note that many redox active chelates have this property. This is thought to facilitate the reaction of substances such as hydrogen peroxide with the metal ion, by allowing direct contact between the peroxide and the iron. As we will show later, 5-iminodaunomycin forms a much less reactive Fe(III) complex in part because it does not readily displaceable and thus renders iron less accessible.

REDOX PROPERTIES OF THE DOXORUBICIN-IRON COMPLEX

While the fully redox chemistry of the doxorubicin-iron complex has been by no means full described, it has already demonstrated a rich chemistry which offers a range of mechanisms for cell damage.

The doxorubicin-iron complex is not stable, but degrades over a period of hours. We have shown that this is the result of an internal electron transfer in which the drug is oxidized and the iron reduced from Fe(III) to Fe(II) (8). This reaction is slow, with a half time of 40-60 min. The resulting Fe(II) can react with oxygen to yield hydrogen peroxide and with hydrogen peroxide to yield the •OH radical. Daunomycin is much less reactive in this reaction (9). This observation suggested that the side chain was a critical determinant of this reaction.

In doxorubicin, the side chain is a ketol. Ketols are known to readily reduce Fe(III) and Cu(II). This forms the basis for the classic tests for reducing sugars and cortisol, both of which are ketols. The nature of the oxidized drug species produced by this reaction have not been characterized. However, the chemistry of cortisol, which has a similar side chain, has been described.

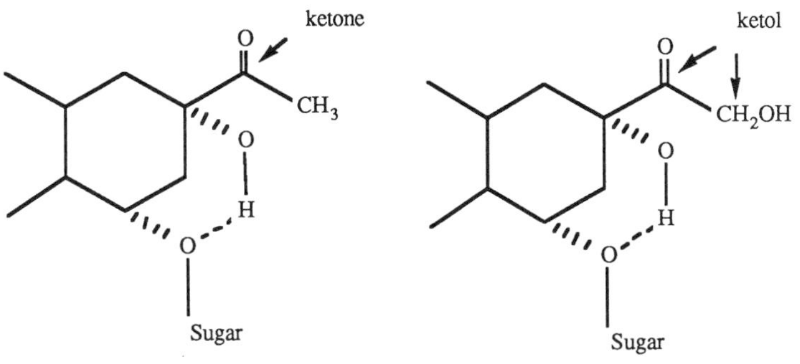

Figure 2. Side chain of doxorubicin compared with daunomycin.

Because Fe(III) is such a common contaminent of laboratory reagents, we think that this chemistry is a major reason for the greater instability of doxorubicin rather than daunorubicin in the laboratory.

The second reaction of interest is the ability of the doxorubicin-iron complex to react with hydrogen peroxide to form •OH. Here also, the drug appears to be the source of the electron needed for this reductive cleavage, although the fate of the drug in this reaction has not been studied. This reaction is markedly stimulated by the addition of DNA (10). This stands in contrast with the inhibitiory effect of DNA addition upon the redox activity of the metal free drug. It is not clear at this time why DNA addition stimulates •OH formation by the doxorubicin-iron complex. One possibility, noted by Floyd (11), is that Fe(II) bound to DNA does not appear to react readily with oxygen, but does still react with hydrogenperoxide. The effect is increased avialability of Fe(II) for •OH formation. It is possible that the doxorubicin bound iron is reduced to Fe(II) in association with DNA, where it is protected from reaction with oxgyen but not hydrogen peroxide.

Finally, the doxorubicin-iron complex catalyzes the reduction of oxygen by thiols. The result is the formation of superoxide, hydrogen peroxide, and •OH radical formation which can result in the oxidative destruction of cell membranes(3). Since this reaction appears to proceed by sequential one electron steps, it is likely that the thiol ts oxidized to its corresponding thiyl radical, although this does not appear to have been studied. The rate of this reaction is much more rapid than the internal electron transfer reaction between doxorubicin and iron. As result, little or no destruction of the doxorubicin-iron complex occurs during this reaction.

ACCESSIBILITY OF IRON *IN VIVO* TO DOXORUBICIN

Because iron is so reactive, most of the iron *in vivo* is held tightly bound. Thus, althought the total cellular iron pool is approximately 0.1 mM, the free iron pool has been estimated to be less than 10^{-11} M. Most of the iron in the cell is stored as ferritin, bound in the porphyrin ring or associated with a range of enzymes such as ribonucleotide reductase. Most of the iron which enters a cell, does so bound to transferrin, the major circulating iron carrier protein. Small amounts of iron can be found associated with various membrane fractions and has been called adventitial iron. However, it is not clear whether or not this is an artifact of procedures used to isolate these subcellular fractions. With this background, it should be clear that it is important to know whether doxorubicin has access to the bound iron pools or whether it is limited to

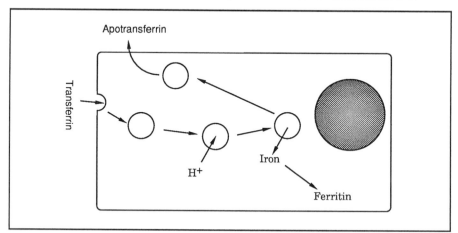

Figure 3 The cellular iron cycle.
"adventitial" iron.

Demant and colleagues (12, 13) have examined the accessibility

of the iron in transferrin. In order to understand this process, it is important to review the outlines of the transferrin cycle (14). Transferrin binds to a specific receptor within the clathrin coated pit complex. After binding to its receptor, it is internalized within a small vesicular structure. The vesicle is then thought to translocate to the perinuclear region. The pH within this vesicle is acidified, and as the pH drops below 6.0, the iron is released. It is not clear at this point how the iron moves from the vesicle to ferritin for storage or to the mitochondria where it is inserted in the porphyrin ring. The vesicle, now containing apotransferrin, migrates back to the cell surface and releases the transferrin into the tissue culture media or extracellular space, as the case may be. Demant and collegues have shown that doxorubicin exhibits a slow rate of release of iron from transferrin at pHs above 7.0. However, this rate increases rapidly as the pH drops below 6.5 with formation of the doxorubicin-iron complex. Thus, the transfer of iron from transferrin to doxorubicin occurs under those conditions that, within the transferrin endocytotic vesicle, would be expected to result in release of iron to the physiologic targets, ferritin or the cytochromes. This would seem to be one of the most likely sites at which doxorubicin might divert iron from its usual metabolic route.

The iron in ferritin is tightly bound in a complex which is encased in multiple ferritin molecules. The geometry of this complex is such that the pores from the outside into the iron containing core are only a few A° in diameter. Thus, while superoxide may gain access to the ferritin core and cause release of iron, many drugs are too large. Demant (15) and Thomas and Aust (16) have shown that doxorubicin will, by itself, cause slow release of iron from ferritin. Thomas and Aust (16) showed that this rate increased dramatically if the doxorubicin was reduced to its semiquinone under anaerobic conditions. Under these conditions, they have reported rapid release of as much as 50% of all of the iron within ferritin.

Under normal conditions, the size of the ferritin iron pool is regulated by iron availability. If iron is entering the cell at a brisk rate, the rate of ferritin matches pace and ferritin bound iron accumulates. If iron is no longer presented to the cell, the ferritin pool depletes itself over 24-48 hours. Although it has not been examined, doxorubicin might have access to the iron as it is released from ferritin.

Thus, although studies have not been done *in vivo* to show that doxorubicin alters cellular ferrokinetics, several sites have been identified where doxorubicin might have access to the large pools of transferrin and ferritin bound iron.

DNA AS A TARGET FOR THE DOXORUBICIN-IRON COMPLEX

The best documented mechanism of DNA binding by the anthracyclines remains intercalation. However, there is ample precedence for another mechanism of DNA binding accessible to hydroxyquinones. One of the major means by which histochemists selectively stain chromatin is through the use of mordant dyes. It should be pointed out that to be useful as a tissue stain, the bond between dye and DNA must be stable enough to survive repeated washing and dehydration through graded alcohol/water mixtures up to absolute alcohol. Many of the dyes used in this process have structures similar the the doxorubicin chromophore. In fact with this historical precedence, it is surprising that

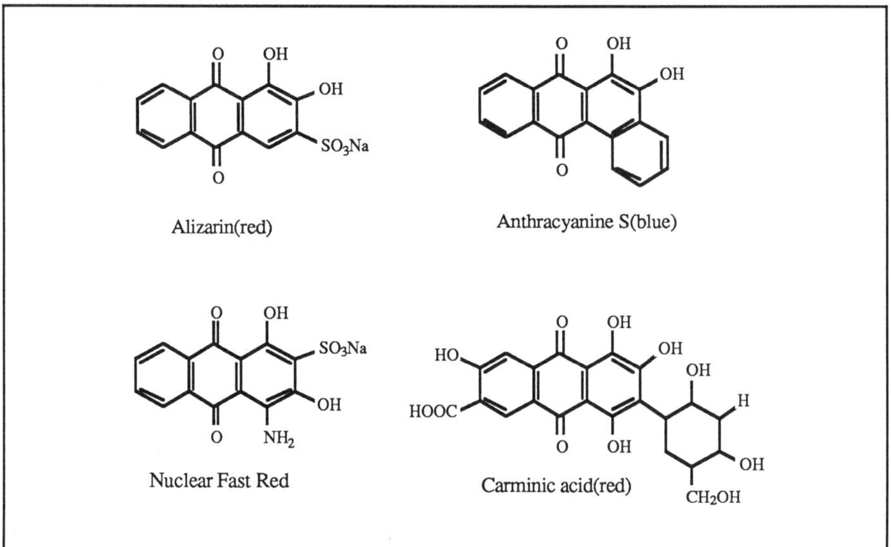

Figure4. Nuclear mordant dyes similar to doxorubicin.

mordant bonding has not been considered as a potential basis for cancer drug development. We have been able to show that the doxorubicin-iron complex binds to DNA to form a ternary drug-iron-DNA complex. This complex appears to be quite stable. We have found that it takes extraction with phenol at 60 °C times two or treatment with SDS and desferal to effectively disrupt the ternary complex. This complex retains much of the redox chemistry of the free drug-iron complex. It reacts with thiols to yield superoxide and hydrogen peroxide (17). As mentioned earlier, it reacts with hydrogen peroxide to yield the •OH radical at a rate more rapid than that seen with the free doxorubicin-iron complex. As a result of these properties, the doxorubicin-iron complex cleaves DNA in the presence of hydrogen peroxide by a process which appears to be at least partially dependent upon •OH formation (10, 18), although participation of a perferyl species can not be ruled out. It should be pointed out that virtually nothing is known about the structure of the doxorubicin-iron-DNA complex.

MEMBRANES AS TARGETS FOR THE DRUG-IRON COMPLEX.

It has long been clear that doxorubicin alters membrane structure and function. There is a detailed literature on this subject, most of it devoted to interactions with with doxorubicin, not the drug-metal complex. We have found that the doxorubicin-iron complex binds tightly to cell membranes with retention of the charge-transfer band at 60 nm characteristic of the doxorubicin-iron complex. In addition, the membrane bound complex retains the capacity to react with exogenous thiols resulting in the oxidative destruction of the membrane. This process includes the formation of superoxide, hydrogen peroxide and the •OH radical. In addition, the drug-metal complex appears to be able to react directly with the membrane without the need of exogenous thiol reducing agents. This results in extensive damage to membrane bound protein thiol groups. It is not clear whether the redox chemistry seen in these experiments without exogenous thiols involves direct oxidation of membrane bound thiols by the drug-metal complex or damage to these thiols secondary to the generation of •OH and other oxyradicals. Oxidation of membrane protein thiols can have catastrophic consequences for membrane function, especially calcium transport (19).

INTERACTION WITH ENZYMATIC DRUG REDOX CYCLING

It is now clear that enzymatic reduction of doxorubicin to its semiquinone does occur *in vivo* in both normal tissue and some tumors. It is therefore of interest to speculate on the potential interactions between the chemistry of the drug-iron complex and that which follows enzymatic reduction of doxorubicin to its semiquinone. First, the drug-iron complex does not, itself, appear to undergo reduction by cytochrome P450 reductase (20). Also, while doxorubicin can generate hydrogen peroxide by reducing directly Fe(III) to Fe(II), the rate of this process is slow relative to the rate of enzymatic reduction to the semiquione and its reaction with oxygen. The direct reduction of Fe(III) by the drug is also slow relative to the reduction of the drug-metal complex via thiols such as glutathione. Given the high concentration of glutathione in cells (>10 mM), it seems likely that this reaction will be rapid *in vivo*. The doxorubicin-iron complex does appear to be an effective catalyst of •OH formation from hydrogen peroxide. Thus, in solution, the dominant sources of hydrogen peroxide generation are likely to be from enzymatic reduction of the drug to its semiquinone and from glutathione dependent reduction of the doxorubicin-iron complex. The conversion of hydrogen peroxide to •OH can occur via two pathways: reductive cleavage of hydrogen peroxide by the drug semiquinone or by the drug-metal complex. Because •OH is so reactive, it is much more effective if generated close to the target. Thus, because the drug-iron complex retains its capacity to generate •OH when bound to membranes or DNA, it is likely to be more efficient in causing damage for a given rate of •OH generation. This may explain the common observation that while the semiquinone can clearly generate •OH in the absence of iron, lipid peroxidation in subcellular organelles is generally iron dependent(21-23). Thus, one potential way in which the two systems may operate would be that the enzymatic reduction of doxorubicin to its semiquinone would generate hydrogen peroxide which could then diffuse to doxorubicin-iron complex bound to critical targets such as the membrane or DNA. The peroxide would react with the bound drug-metal complex resulting in local generation of •OH and destruction of the target. Because production of •OH in free solution is likely to be much less efficient in causing damage, just removal of iron from the system would markedly lessen injury. However, the protection would not be complete because •OH can still be generated by the drug semiquinone. This process can, however, be modulated by increased removal of hydrogen peroxide. Thus, increased expression of either catalase or glutathione peroxidase combined with iron chelation should provide additive protection. We have noted increased expression of glutathione peroxidase in doxorubicin resistant human breast cancer cells.

ROLE OF DOXORUBICIN-FE(III) IN CARDIAC INJURY

There is no direct evidence that the doxorubicin-iron complex is involved in cardiac injury. There is, however, evidence that iron itself plays a role in both the cardiac toxicity and lipid peroxidation in heart muscle. Several workers have shown that iron is required for doxorubicin-induced lipid peroxidation in cardiac subcellular organelles (22,23). In addition, there is a good correlation between the cardiac toxicity of a range of anthracycline analogs and the redox activity of their iron complexes (24). However, the most interesting observation is that ICRF-187, an EDTA derivative, is able to block cardiac toxicity in both animals and

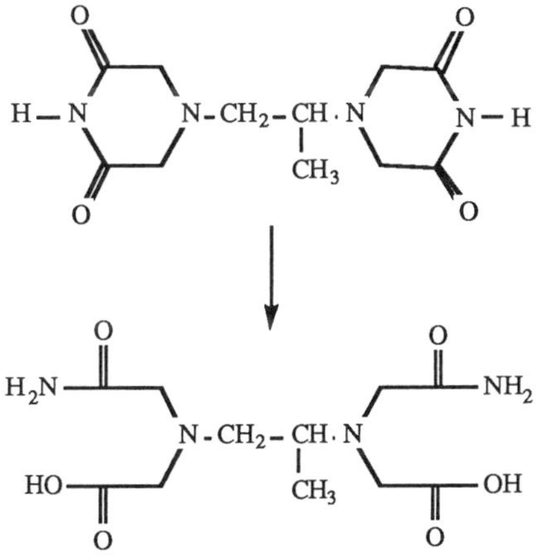

man (24,25).

Figure 5. The hydrolysis of ICRF-187 to the putative chelating species.

In ICRF-187, the dicarboxylic acid chelating groups have been replaced with an amide ring. The result is a nonpolar compound which should enter cells much more readily. Clinical trials with this compound have shown that it is an effective iron chelator in man, resulting in a 10 fold increase in urinary iron clearance (25). The parent compound is not a very good iron chelator. However, ICRF-187 undergoes hydrolysis to yield the corresponding acid amine which would be a good chelator of Fe(II). We have previously shown that Fe(II) chelators efficiently shut down the redox cycle of the doxorubicin-iron complex (8). The hydrolysis of ICRF-187 will be pH dependent and so the formation of the putative chelating species should occur more rapidly in normal tissue than in acidic tumor cells. This may, in part, explain why ICFR-197 prevents cardiac toxicity without altering the effectiveness of doxorubicin against breast cancer. Based upon the structure of ICRF-187, its proven activity as an iron chelator in man, and the chemistry of its hydrolysis products, it seems that iron chelation must be viewed as its most likely mechanism of action. This hypothesis, however, remains to be tested.

IMPLICATIONS FOR ANALOG DEVELOPMENT

Can anthracyclines be produced which lack the redox chemistry of the doxorubicin-iron complex but which retain antitumor activity? We have examined a range of chromophore analogs of doxorubicin and found that the anthracyclines which lacked iron chelating ability lacked both antitumor activity and cardiac toxicity (24). We have recently examined the iron chemistry of 5-iminodaunomycin and have found this drug to have unique properties relevent to this issue (26). This drug is neither cardiotoxic nor mutagenic. While it exhibits antitumor activity, its potency in some cell lines is less than that of doxorubicin. We have found that it is even a better chelator of Fe(III) than is doxorubicin and will abstract iron from the doxorubicin-iron complex. However, the 5-iminodaunomycin complex is much less active than doxorubicin in the reductive cleavage of hydrogen peroxide to $\bullet OH$. In addition, it is much less active in catalyzing the hydrogen peroxide dependent cleavage of DNA. These properties seem to be the result of two factors. First, it does not participate in the internal electron transfer by which doxorubicin reduces the bound Fe(III) to Fe(II). Second, it chelates Fe(III) so tightly that the metal ion is no longer accessible to solvent water and therefore presumably hydrogen peroxide. This results show that their exist anthracycline structures which can function as effective iron chelators without the complications which result from the redox activity seen with doxorubicin. It should be noted that 5-iminodaunomycin does cause topoisomerase II associated DNA cleavage as well. This demonstrates that it is possible to cleanly dissociate the redox biochemistry of the anthracyclines from the consequences of DNA intercalation. Further analog development in this direction with an eye toward increased potency may be of value.

REFERENCES
1.   Calendi, E., Di Marco, A., Reggiani, M., Scarpinato, B., Valentina, L. (1965) Biochem. Biophys. Acta. 103: 25-49.
2.   Spiro, T.G., Allerton, F.E., Renner, J., Tergis, R. Bils, R. and Sallaman, P. (1966) J. Am. Chem. Soc. 88, 12-19.
3.   Myers, C.E., Gianni, L., Simone, C.B., Klecker, R. and Greene, R. (1982) Biochem. 21:1707-1713.
4.   Gianni, L., Zweier, J.L., Levy, A., and Myers, C.E. (1985) J. Biol. Chem. 260: 6820-6826.
5.   Gianni, L., Corden, B. and Myers, C.E. (1983) In: Reviews in Biochemical Toxicology eds. Hodgson, E., Bend, J.R., Philpot, R.M. (Elsevier), pp 1-83.
6.   May, P., Williams, G.N., and Williams, D. R. (1980) Eur. J. Cancer 16: 1275-1276.
7.   Zweier, J., Gianni, L., Muindi, J., and Myers, C.E. (1986) Biochem. Biophys. Acta. 884: 326-336.
8.   Muindi, J.R.F., Sinha, B.K., Gianni, L. and Myers, C.E. (1984) FEBS Lett. 172: 226-230.
9.   Floyd, R.A., and Lewis, C.A. (1983) Biochem. 22: 2645-2649.
10.   Demant, E.J.F., and Norskov-Lauritsen, N. (1986) FEBS Lett. 196: 321-323.
11.   Princiotto, J.V. and Zapolsi, E.J. (1975) Nature 255: 87-88.
12.   Carver, F.J. and Frieden, E. (1978) Biochem. 17: 167-172.
13.   Van Renswoude, J. Bridges, K.R., Harford, J.B. and Klausner, R.D. (1982) Proc. Natl. Acad. Sci. USA. 79: 6186-6190.
14.   Yamashiro, D.J., Tycko, B., Fluss, S.R. and Maxfield, F. R. (1984) Cell 37: 789-800.
15.   Demant, E.J.F. (1984) FEBS Lett. 176:97-100.
16.   Thomas, C. E., and Aust, S. D. (1986) Arch. Biochem. Biophys. 248: 684-689.
17.   Eliot, H., Gianni, L. and Myers, C. E. (1984) Biochem. 23: 928-936.

18. Jones, D. P., Thor, H., Smith, M.T., Jewell, S.A. and Orrenius, S. (1983) J. Biol. Chem. 258: 6390-6393.
19. Beraldo, H. Garnier-Suillerot, A., Tosi, L. and Lavelle, F. (1985) Biochem. 24: 284-289.
20. Mimnaugh, E. G., Gram, E.G., Trush, M.A. (1983) J. Pharmacol. Exp. Ther. 226: 806-816.
21. Mimnaugh, E. G., Trush, M.A., and Gram, T. E. (1983) Cancer Treat Rep. 67: 731-736.
22. Doroshow, J. H. (1983) Cancer Res. 43: 4543-4551.
23. Muindi, J.R.F., Sinha, B.K., Gianni, L., and Myers, C.E. (1985) Mol. Pharmacol. 27: 356-365.
24. Herman, E. H., Ferrans, V.J., Myers, C.E. and Van Vleet, J.F. (1985) Cancer Res. 45: 276-281.
25. Von Hoff, D.D., Howser, D., Lewis, B.J., Holchenberg, J., Weiss, R.B. and Young, R.C. (1981) Cancer Treat. Rep. 65: 249-252.
26. Myers, C.E., Muindi, J.R.F., Zweier, J. and Sinha, B. K. (1987) J. Biol. Chem. in press.

Role of Reactive Oxygen Production in Doxorubicin Cardiac Toxicity
J.H. Doroshow

INTRODUCTION

Doxorubicin and related anthracycline quinones play a central role in the chemotherapeutic management of acute myelogenous leukemia, the non-Hodgkin's lymphomas, and carcinomas of the breast, lung, and thyroid (1). The clinical usefulness of these drugs may, however, be compromised by the development of a dose-related, congestive cardiomyopathy that is sometimes fatal (2). Over the past decade, a substantial body of experimental data has been published which supports the hypothesis that the myocardial injury produced by anthracycline antibiotics is related to drug-induced reactive oxygen production in the heart (3-6). These investigations include studies which show that the morphologic expression of doxorubicin cardiac toxicity may be enhanced by inhibition of cardiac antioxidant defense systems; that damage to the heart may be reduced or abolished by pretreatment of experimental animals with various free radical scavengers; and that cyclical reduction and oxidation of the doxorubicin quinone leads to the depletion of critical cardiac energy stores, as well as to the inability of intact myocytes to maintain calcium homeostasis (7-10).

To understand the role of free radical formation in the pathogenesis of this syndrome, this study will review the sites and mechanisms of doxorubicin-stimulated oxygen radical metabolism in the heart and the potential for toxicity produced by drug-related oxyradical formation in each cardiac organelle.

MATERIALS AND METHODS

Materials

Male 200-250 g Sprague-Dawley rats were obtained from Simonsen Laboratories, Gilroy, CA and housed on hardwood bedding with access to feed and water ad libitum. Fresh bovine hearts were a gift of the Gold Star Meat Co., Los Angeles, CA. Doxorubicin hydrochloride was purchased from Adria Laboratories, Inc., Wilmington, Del. Daunorubicin, 5-iminodaunorubicin, and menogaril were supplied by the Drug Synthesis and Chemistry Branch, Division of Cancer Treatment, National Cancer Institute, Bethesda, MD. Cytochrome c, dimethyl sulfoxide (DMSO), horse heart myoglobin, hyaluronidase (type I-S), and bovine erythrocyte superoxide dismutase (SOD, 2900 units/mg) were from Sigma Chemical Co, St. Louis, MO. Deferoxamine mesylate was purchased from CIBA Pharmaceutical Co., Summit, NJ. Collagenase (type II) was obtained from Cooper Biomedical Inc., Freehold, NJ. Catalase of analytical grade (65,000 unis/mg) was purchased from Boehringer Mannheim Biochemicals, Indianapolis, IN, and was devoid of SOD activity.

Methods

Cardiac subcellular fractions from rat heart (11), or bovine heart (12) were prepared by previously described techniques. Viable, beating adult rat heart myocytes were prepared from minced ventricular muscle as previously described (13) except that intact cells were separated from damaged myocytes by metrizamide density centrifugation (14). Typically, the viable cell yield, determined by the presence of rod-shaped morphology and exclusion of 0.1% trypan blue dye, ranged from 70-80%.

Superoxide anion production was determined by the rate of SOD-inhibitable acetylated cytochrome c reduction (11); oxygen consumption was measured at 37°C with a YSI model 53 oxygen monitoring system by our previously published technique (11); and the formation of a strong oxidizing species with the chemical characteristics of the hydroxyl radical was detected by measurement of CH_4 production from DMSO by gas chromatography (12).

RESULTS

Oxygen radical production by cardiac mitochondria

Since mitochondria are a major intracellular site of
anthracycline cardiac toxicity, drug-enhanced oxygen radical
formation was studied in beef heart submitochondrial particles
(BH-SMP). As previously demonstrated by Thayer (3), our
investigations revealed that doxorubicin dramatically increased
the rate of superoxide anion production by BH-SMP (Table 1).
Furthermore, related anthracyclines, such as daunorubicin, also
significantly increased superoxide formation by BH-SMP. However,
when the anthracycline quinone moiety is blocked by an imine
substitution, electron transfer to molecular oxygen was significantly diminished (Table 1). Reactive oxygen production in
BH-SMP required NADH; in related studies employing inhibitors of
the mitochondrial electron transport chain, as well as reverse
electron flow, complex I was found to be the major site of
reduction of the anthracycline quinone by BH-SMP (15).

In addition to a dose-dependent increase in superoxide anion
formation, related experiments revealed that under similar
experimental conditions anthracycline treatment of BH-SMP produced
a significant increase in CH_4 generation from DMSO (Table 2).
Hydroxyl radical production in this setting was confirmed by the
competitive inhibition of drug-induced CH_4 formation by known
scavengers of the hydroxyl radical and by the inhibitory effects
of SOD and catalase but not the heat-denatured enzymes (Table 2).
These experiments were performed with buffers treated with Chelex
100 resin to remove adventitial iron from the reaction mixtures
(12); however, despite this precaution, drug-stimulated
hydroxyl radical production was significantly reduced in the
presence of deferoxamine, a chelating agent which binds iron in
a fashion that makes it unavailable as a catalyst for hydroxyl
radical formation from hydrogen peroxide (12). Hence, these
studies suggest that membrane-associated iron or iron proteins
may be proximal catalysts for hydroxyl radical formation by
BH-SMP.

Table 1. Anthracycline-enhanced superoxide production (11,12).

Reaction system	Sarcoplasmic reticulum	Beef heart submito-chondrial particles
	$nmol \cdot min^{-1} \cdot mg^{-1}$	
Control	1.4 ± 0.2[a]	1.6 ± 0.2
Doxorubicin		
25 µM	2.2 ± 0.1[b]	32 ± 1.2[b]
90 µM	5.6 ± 0.5[b]	70 ± 2.7[b]
Doxorubicin (135 µM)	9.0 ± 0.7[b]	85 ± 3.2[b]
minus NADH	-	0
minus NADPH	0	-
using heat-denatured membranes	0	0
Daunorubicin		
90 µM	-	32 ± 1.5[b]
135 µM	9.1 ± 0.4[b]	-
5-Iminodaunorubicin		
90 µM	-	4.8 ± 2.0
135 µM	1.9 ± 0.4	-

[a]Mean ± S.E. of 3-7 independent experiments.
[b]$p < 0.05$ compared to control.

Reactive oxygen production by the cardiac sarcotubular system

Anthracycline cardiac toxicity in man and in experimental animal models is associated with a characteristic dilatation and breakdown of sarcotubular membranes (16). Because of this morphologic picture, as well as the importance of the sarco-tubular system in the maintenance of myocardial calcium homeostasis, drug-stimulated reactive oxygen production was measured in cardiac sarcoplasmic reticulum. As shown in Table 1, treatment with doxorubicin significantly increased superoxide anion production in heart sarcoplasmic reticular membranes in a process that was drug dose- and NADPH-dependent. In analogy to studies with BH-SMP, 5-iminodaunorubicin did not significantly increase superoxide production by sarcotubular membranes. As

Table 2. Stimulation of hydroxyl radical formation in heart mitochondria by anthracyclines (12).

Experimental system	Methane production
	nmol/30 min
Control	0
Doxorubicin 20 μM	0.4 ± 0.1[a,b]
Doxorubicin 90 μM	1.4 ± 0.1[b]
minus NADH	0
minus DMSO	0
using heat-denatured mitochondria	0
plus catalase (1500 u/ml)	0[c]
plus heat-denatured catalase	1.5 ± 0.05[b]
plus SOD (20 μg/ml)	0.3 ± 0.02[c]
plus heat-denatured SOD	1.4 ± 0.04[b]
Doxorubicin 135 μM	2.2 ± 0.25[b]
plus N-acetylcysteine (50 mM)	0.2 ± 0.03[c]
plus thiourea (50 mM)	0.04 ± 0.02[c]
plus deferoxamine (50 μM)	0.23 ± 0.02[c]
Daunorubicin 90 μM	0.74 ± 0.03[b]
5-Iminodaunorubicin 90 μM	0.11 ± 0.01[c]

[a] mean ± S.E. of 3 to 6 experiments.
[b] $p < 0.05$ compared to control.
[c] $p < 0.05$ compared to sample containing doxorubicin alone.

previously reported (11), superoxide anion formation was accompanied by a dose-related oxidation of NADPH and was significantly decreased by inhibitors of NADPH cytochrome P-450 reductase. These studies suggest that NADPH cytochrome P-450 reductase activity associated with cardiac sarcoplasmic reticulum is the enzyme responsible for anthracycline reduction at this site.

We have also found that the anthracycline antibiotics enhance hydroxyl radical production by cardiac sarcoplasmic reticulum (17). However, this system, in contrast to BH-SMP, requires the addition of iron or iron proteins to stimulate hydroxyl radical formation. In this setting, cardiac ferritin as well as iron-saturated transferrin and oxymyoglobin are potent catalysts of CH_4 production from DMSO by anthracycline-treated cardiac sarcoplasmic reticulum.

Anthracycline-enhanced oxyradical formation by cardiac cytoplasmic proteins

Rat heart cytosol contains a heat-labile factor that in the presence of NADH is capable of supporting doxorubicin-enhanced superoxide production (11). Superoxide anion formation in heart cytosol increased from 0.56 ± 0.20 to 6.22 ± 0.67 nmol· min^{-1}· mg^{-1} after addition of 135 µM doxorubicin. Superoxide production was inhibited 35% by addition of 100 µM allopurinol suggesting that xanthine dehydrogenase activity may, in part, be responsible for drug reduction in heart cytoplasm.

Recent studies from our laboratory have revealed a second source of potential drug reducing activity in myocyte cytoplasm. We have shown that electron transfer from cardiac oxymyoglobin to the anthracycline quinone yields reduced oxygen species; as measured by the production of adrenochrome from epinephrine in the presence of oxymyoglobin and deferoxamine, doxorubicin at concentrations of 50 or 135 µM increased adrenochrome formation from undetectable control levels to 11.7 ± 2.9 or 22.0 ± 7.3 nmol/60 min (18).

Oxygen consumption by intact rat heart myocytes treated with anthracyclines.

To determine whether the stimulation of reactive oxygen production by anthracyclines could be demonstrated with intact cells as well as subcellular fractions, we examined the effect of anthracycline antibiotics on cyanide-resistant respiration by beating cardiac myocytes obtained from adult rats (19). As shown in Table 3, doxorubicin and related anthracyclines produced a dose-dependent increase in myocyte oxygen consumption. At a doxorubicin concentration of 400 µM, cyanide-resistant respiration exceeded the normal rate of electron flow in control myocytes. Doxorubicin-enhanced oxygen consumption was accompanied by the

Table 3. Effect of anthracyclines on oxygen consumption by rat heart myocytes (19).

Reaction system	Oxygen consumption
	nmol· min^{-1}· 2 x 10^6 cells^{-1}
Control	5.40 ± 0.40[a]
+ KCN (5 mM)	1.00 ± 0.10
Doxorubicin + KCN (5 mM)	
10 µM	1.40 ± 0.01[b]
90 µM	2.84 ± 0.35[b]
Doxorubicin (400 µM) + KCN (5 mM)	5.74 ± 0.28[b]
plus catalase (2500 units/ml)	3.65 ± 0.06[c]
Menogaril (400 µM) + KCN (5 mM)	2.57 ± 0.06[b]
5-Iminodaunorubicin (400 µM)	
+ KCN (5 mM)	1.24 ± 0.24

[a] mean ± S.E. of 3 to 5 experiments.
[b] $p < 0.05$ compared to corresponding control.
[c] $p < 0.05$ compared to sample containing doxorubicin alone.

formation of hydrogen peroxide. After treatment with 400 µM doxorubicin, hydrogen peroxide production increased from undetectable control levels to 1.30 ± 0.02 nmol· min^{-1}· 10^7 myocytes, $p < 0.01$. Thus, treatment of cardiac myocytes with doxorubicin stimulates an oxidation-reduction cycle capable of overwhelming cardiac antioxidant defenses in the intact cell.

DISCUSSION

In these experiments, we have demonstrated that anthracycline antibiotics increase the rate of oxygen consumption and hydrogen peroxide production of adult cardiac myocytes. Studies using cardiac subcellular fractions suggest that oxyradical production by intact cells can be explained by redox cycling of the anthracycline quinone at complex I of the mitochondrial electron transport chain, and by reaction of the drug with the NADPH cytochrome P-450 reductase activity associated with cardiac sarcoplasmic reticulum, and with the xanthine dehydrogenase and oxymyoglobin found in the cytoplasm of heart myocytes.

Since heart mitochondria occupy 35% of the total myocardial cell volume, which is approximately 10 times that of the sarcotubular system (20), drug-related reactive oxygen production by cardiac mitochondria may play a significant role in the cardiac toxicity of the anthracycline antibiotics. Thus, electron flow from NADH-linked substrates directly to oxygen through the anthracycline quinone (rather than via cytochrome oxidase) significantly decreases cellular ATP production (9) while generating toxic oxygen species capable of damaging the mitochondrial calcium pump (21) as well as mitochondrial membrane integrity. Hydrogen peroxide produced by the mitochondrial metabolism of the anthracyclines may also contribute to drug-induced hydroxyl radical production at other cellular locales.

As we have recently demonstrated (10), calcium sequestration by cardiac sarcoplasmic reticulum is inhibited significantly by enzymatically-initiated redox cycling of the doxorubicin quinone. Since the sarcotubular calcium pump plays the major role in regulating intracellular calcium concentration in the heart, our studies suggest that oxyradical-related alterations in calcium sequestration produced by anthracyclines could be intimately involved in the depression of contraction-coupling, and hence depressed cardiac output, in patients treated with anthracyclines.

We have also shown that the cytoplasmic compartment of myocardial cells is exposed to a free radical flux generated by anthracycline antibiotics. Direct damage to myofibrillar proteins could be produced by this mechanism. Finally, the oxidation of oxymyoglobin by anthracyclines, in addition to contributing to cytoplasmic oxygen radical formation, leads to a loss of oxygen carrying capacity in the myocyte, since reduction of the metmyoglobin formed by this reaction is limited by the inhibitory effect of doxorubicin on cardiac metmyoglobin reductase (22).

In summary, anthracycline antibiotics stimulate an oxygen radical cascade by several different mechanisms throughout cardiac myocytes. Toxic effects of the strongly oxidizing species that are produced include inhibition of mitochondrial ATP production and the sarcotubular calcium pump, as well as oxyradical-related changes in membrane integrity. The widespread nature of the reactive oxygen formation produced by anthracyclines in the heart and the critical functions impaired by these reactions strongly suggest that redox cycling of the anthracycline quinone plays an important part in the cardiac toxicity of these drugs.

ACKNOWLEDGMENTS

I wish to thank Sunny Ilagan-Aure for her skilled secretarial assistance. This study was supported by grant CA 31788 from the National Cancer Institute and by a scholarship from the Leukemia Society of America.

REFERENCES

1. Young, R.C., Ozols, R.F. and Myers, C.E. (1981) N. Eng. J. Med. 305: 139-153.
2. Lenaz, L. and Page, J. (1976) Cancer Treat. Rev. 3: 111-120.
3. Thayer, W.S. (1977) Chem.-Biol. Interact. 19: 265-278.
4. Bachur, N.R., Gordon, S.L. and Gee, M.W. (1977) Mol. Pharmacol. 13: 901-910.
5. Revis, N.W. and Marusic, N. (1978) J. Mol. Cell. Cardiol. 10: 945-951.
6. Myers, C.E., McGuire, W.P., Liss, R.H., Ifrim, I., Grotzinger, K. and Young, R.C. (1977) Science 197: 165-167.
7. Doroshow, J.H., Locker, G.Y. and Myers, C.E. (1980) J. Clin. Invest. 65: 128-135.
8. Doroshow, J.H., Locker, G.Y., Ifrim, I. and Myers, C.E. (1981) J. Clin. Invest. 68: 1058-1064.
9. Davies, K.J.A., Doroshow, J.H. and Hochstein, P. (1983) FEBS Lett. 153: 227-230.
10. Harris, R.N. and Doroshow, J.H. (1985) Biochem. Biophys. Res. Commun. 130: 739-745.
11. Doroshow, J.H. (1983) Cancer Res. 43: 460-472.
12. Doroshow, J.H. and Davies, K.J.A. (1986) J. Biol. Chem. 261: 3068-3074.
13. Glick, M.R., Burns, A.H. and Reddy, W.J. (1974) Analyt. Biochem. 61: 32-42.
14. Wittenberg, B.A. and Robinson, T.F. (1981) Cell and Tissue Res. 216: 231-251.
15. Davies, K.J.A. and Doroshow, J.H. (1986) J. Biol. Chem. 261: 3060-3067.
16. Ferrans, V.J. (1978) Cancer Treat. Rep. 62: 955-961.
17. Doroshow, J.H. (1983) Proc. Amer. Assoc. Cancer Res. 24: 255.
18. Doroshow, J.H. (1987) Proc. Amer. Assoc. Cancer Res. 28: 262.
19. Doroshow, J.H. (1986) Proc. Amer. Assoc. Cancer Res. 27: 250.

20. Page, E. and McCallister, L.P. (1973) Am. J. Cardiol. 31: 172-181.
21. Harris, E.J., Booth, R. and Cooper, M.B. (1982) FEBS Lett. 146: 267-270.
22. Taylor, D. and Hochstein, P. (1978) Biochem. Pharmacol. 27: 2079-2082.

Adriamycin Cardiac Toxicity — An Assessment of Approaches to Cardiac Monitoring and Cardioprotection

R.S. Benjamin, S.P. Chawla, M.S. Ewer,
G.N. Hortobagyi, B. Mackay, S.S. Legha,
C.H. Carrasco, and S. Wallace

Adriamycin is one of the most effective chemotherapeutic agents in the treatment of a broad spectrum of malignancies. The initial discovery that its prolonged use could lead to progressive, refractory, irreversible and almost uniformly fatal congestive heart failure has been a major impediment to its more widespread use in the curative treatment of early cancer and to prolonging its use in responding patients with advanced disease.

The most important contribution to minimizing adriamycin-induced congestive heart failure (CHF) was the discovery of its cumulative-dose relationship by Gottlieb and associates (1, 2). Maximum cumulative doses of 600 mg/m^2, then 550 mg/m^2, and most recently 450 mg/m^2 have been recommended for adriamycin administration. Von Hoff, in an analysis of risk factors for development of congestive heart failure, plotted the cumulative incidence of CHF vs total dose and confirmed both the increased incidence above 450 mg/m^2 and the still greater risk at higher doses. He also suggested a low level of toxicity at doses traditionally considered safe (3). Minow and associates pointed out that with cumulative-dose limitation, if heart failure occurred more than 3 weeks after the last adriamycin dose, it was less likely to be fatal (2). This was the first suggestion that adriamycin cardiomyopathy might be reversible (2). A more recent analysis by Haq et al, shows that the majority of adults who develop adriamycin-induced CHF respond to standard treatment and often recover fully (4).

Cardiac Monitoring

The improved prognosis of patients with adriamycin cardiac toxicity is primarily due to clinical awareness of the problem and to cumulative-dose limitation. Improvements in cardiac monitoring, utilizing determination of cardiac ejection fraction (EF), by nuclear cineangiography or echocardiography, and direct endomyo-cardial biopsies have increased the quantification of drug-induced cardiac damage, permitting the study of less toxic approaches to drug administration, and in some cases, to individualization of therapy. The most important monitoring tool in our research has been the endomyocardial biopsy.

The description by Billingham and collaborators that specific abnormalities could be detected after adriamycin administration in small pieces of cardiac muscle, easily obtainable by endomyocardial biopsy, is of tremendous importance (5, 6). The biopsy allows direct observation of the target organ for toxicity. The morpho-logic abnormalities can be detected after cumulative adriamycin doses far below those required to produce congestive heart failure. The pathologic findings include vacuolization produced by swelling of the sarcoplasmic reticulum, myofibrillar dropout, and necrosis. These findings, although ultimately visible by light microscopy, can be detected in most cases only by the electron microscope (EM).

Although we found the initial Billingham grading system somewhat difficult to quantify, we were tremendously impressed by the

correlation between cardiac biopsy grade and cumulative dose. After
learning how to estimate biopsy grade according to the Billingham
system, we modified the grading system to a half-point scale using a
more easily quantitative approach (Table 1) (7).

Table 1. Mackay Scale for Grading Endomyocardial Biopsies*

	Average Number of Muscle Cells per Block Demonstrating the Following Abnormalities Based on EM Evaluation of at Least 6 Blocks		
		Myofibrillar	
Grade	Vacuoles	Dropout	Necrosis
0.5	<4	0	0
1	4-10	<3	0
1.5	>10	3-5	<2
2	-	6-8	2-5
3	-	>8	>5

* Modified from Mackay, et al (7)

The final biopsy grade was determined after evaluation of at
least 6 EM blocks based on the average number of muscle cells per
block showing each of the 3 morphologic abnormalities related to
adriamycin. Necrosis was considered to have worse prognostic
implications than myofibrillar dropout, which was considered more
serious than vacuolization. The presence of necrosis, even in a
single cell, was enough to grade the biopsy as 1.5. Similarly, any
myofibrillar dropout made the biopsy at least grade 1. A few
vacuoles per block in the absence of other abnormalities were
considered minor; thus the biopsy was graded as 0.5.

In addition, the biopsy was graded according to the worst abnormality present. For example, the number of cells showing myofibrillar dropout for a grade 1 biopsy should be less than 3 per block, and the number of cells showing vacuolization for a grade 1 biopsy should be 4-10. If a biopsy showed either one of those abnormalities, it would be graded as grade 1. If the biopsy showed both of those abnormalities, the biopsy grade was automatically raised to 1.5 (7, 8).

During assessment of new approaches to decreasing the cardiac toxicity of adriamycin, patients were monitored every 4 courses of chemotherapy with endomyocardial biopsy, and every 2 courses of therapy with nuclear cardiac ejection fraction. Since the mean cardiac biopsy grade at a cumulative adriamycin dose of 450 mg/m^2, our previous cutoff point, was 1.8, we elected to continue treatment until a grade 2 biopsy or evidence of CHF. Two hundred fifty-two patients who received more than 500 mg/m^2 of adriamycin were evaluated during these studies with 411 endomyocardial biopsies and 1063 cardiac scans for EF determination. We reviewed the outcome of these patients to determine the effectiveness of the monitoring program (9, 10). Seventy-two patients were eventually diagnosed with CHF, which was fatal in only two patients.

When the highest biopsy grade was 0 to 0.5, the risk of developing CHF after up to 4 additional courses of adriamycin was only about 2%. When the biopsy was grade 1, the risk of developing heart failure was only 5%. When the biopsy grade was 1.5 or higher, however, the risk of developing CHF was almost 25%. When adriamycin was stopped because of a grade 2 cardiac biopsy, the risks of heart failure were actually less than when the adriamycin was continued and the biopsy grade was 1.5. Thus, our initial decision to treat to a grade 2 biopsy has been revised, and we now treat only to a grade 1.5 biopsy. Any cardiac biopsy of grade 1.5 or higher is considered "high-grade."

Cardiac ejection fraction varies substantially from institution to institution in our experience. For that reason, we evaluated only the cardiac ejection fractions performed at M. D. Anderson Hospital. The mean baseline EF was 72%, somewhat higher than in other institutions. The cardiac EF was considered to be normal as long as it was above 60%. Lower ejection fractions were accompanied by a note of caution and recommendation of cardiac consultation (for possible endomyocardial biopsy) should further adriamycin be considered. In fact, however, the risk of developing CHF with up to 2 additional treatment courses was identical, 12%, for those with "abnormal" EF's between 55% and 59%, and for those with "normal" EF's between 60% and 64%. The risk of development of heart failure was 14% for those with ejection fractions of 50% and 54%. This group with intermediate EF's of 50-64% represented 36% of our patients.

Patients whose ejection fraction was 65% or higher, had only a 5% risk of developing CHF, equivalent to that of patients with a grade 1 cardiac biopsy. In contrast, those few whose ejection fractions were 45-49% had a 25% risk of developing CHF, and those with EF's below 45% had a 40% risk of developing CHF. Thus, by EF grouping there is a high-risk group with EF's below 50%, a low risk group, with EF's above 65%, and an intermediate group with EF's ranging from 50%-64%.

Alexander and associates have suggested that the change in ejection fraction from baseline may be of greater prognostic importance than the absolute EF and have emphasized that patients who go on to develop CHF first have a decrease in EF of more than 15 percentage points to a value less than 45% (11). They have termed this "moderately severe" cardiac toxicity. The risk of developing heart failure by fall in EF is shown for our patients in Table 2.

Table 2. Risk of Developing CHF by Decrease in Ejection Fraction

| | Fall in Ejection Fraction (Absolute Percentage Points) | | | |
	<5	6-10	11-15	>15
Number of Patients	92	64	23	25
Percent Developing CHF	10	6	9	16

The overall risk of developing CHF was 16% for those with >15 percentage point fall in cardiac EF, only a very slight, statistically insignificant increase in risk compared with those with lesser EF changes. For patients with a >15 point fall in ejection fraction whose last EF was $\geq$ 50%, the risk of developing CHF was only 11%. In contrast, it was 29% for those whose lowest EF was below 50%. There were 2 patients whose lowest EF was <50%, but who did not have a 15 point fall in EF. Both developed CHF. Thus, from our point of view, the absolute value of the lowest EF is of greater prognostic value than the degree of fall in predicting the development of CHF.

Cardiac ejection fractions are very helpful in determining if adriamycin can be safely continued (>65%) or should be discontinued (<50%), but are not helpful for the intermediate group of patients whose cardiac EF is between 50% and 64%. We have looked at exercise-induced increments or decrements in EF to determine whether we could identify patients within this group who were at higher risk of developing heart failure (12). Unfortunately, we could determine no benefit from the ability to increase EF with exercise, and no increased risk from the lack of such ability.

Only the cardiac biopsy was helpful in differentiating high-risk patients from low-risk patients in the intermediate EF group. For those with low-grade biopsies (grade 0-1), the risk of developing CHF was 4% with continued adriamycin. In contrast, for those with high-grade biopsies ($\geq$ grade 1.5), the risk of developing heart failure was 33%. It should be emphasized, however, that all of these patients received higher cumulative doses of adriamycin than those usually recommended. Once appropriate cumulative-dose limitation can be determined, the necessity of cardiac monitoring decreases substantially. While actively studying methods to ameliorate adriamycin cardiac toxicity and extend the cumulative doses administered, we performed 2 endomyocardial biopsies each day. Now that appropriate cumulative doses have been determined for the adriamycin schedules which we utilize most frequently, we perform only about 1 cardiac biopsy for adriamycin toxicity every 2 months.

Cardioprotection

Attempts to decrease cardiac toxicity have included schedule manipulation, analogue development, and co-administration of putative cardioprotective agents. The initial testing of adriamycin employed a variety of schedules of administration, which appeared to have equivalent therapeutic effects but differing patterns of acute toxicity (13). There was more prominent mucositis in schedules utilizing multiple daily injections or courses repeated more frequently than every 3 weeks (14). Clinical pharmacology studies demonstrated that adriamycin had a long plasma half-life, and it was suggested that a single-dose every 3 weeks would be pharmacologically rational (15, 16). Either because of the scientific rationale or the practical simplicity of a single-dose schedule, the majority of regimens have utilized single-dose administration every 3 weeks, hereafter referred to as the standard schedule.

Weiss from the Central Oncology Group was the first to suggest that weekly adriamycin administration at lower doses per injection would decrease cardiac toxicity (17). Perhaps because of the difficulty in clinical assessment of adriamycin cardiac toxicity, this schedule did not gain rapid popularity. A confirmatory report from the Western Cancer Study Group (18), however, and the compilation of data by Von Hoff (3), lead other investigators to re-examine the question of weekly adriamycin administration. Our study, reported by Valdivieso et al (19), and the study of Torti (20) at Stanford both utilized endomyocardial biopsies and confirmed without question the decreased cardiac toxicity of the weekly schedule. In addition, it should be noted that statistically significant advantages for weekly over 3-weekly adriamycin could be demonstrated with a total of only 35 endomyocardial biopsies, most at low cumulative doses (19), whereas the difference in incidence of CHF required evaluation of hundreds of patients because most went off study with progressive disease before reaching sufficient cumulative doses to put them at risk of heart failure.

The only reasonable explanation for the decreased cardiac toxicity of weekly adriamycin is the decreased peak drug levels in plasma together with time to eliminate the peak before re-exposure of the myocardium to the next dose. Pharmacologically, the best way to decrease peak levels is by prolonging the rate of infusion. Thus, while the "pharmacologically rational" approach to adriamycin administration had initially been a rapid, single, high-dose injection, the pharmacologically rational way of decreasing cardiac toxicity is precisely the opposite.

Realizing the potential of dose-limiting mucositis, we initiated our first study with a 24-hr infusion of single-agent adriamycin at dose of 60 mg/m^2 (21). The protocol was designed with a fixed dose on subsequent courses, but the duration of infusion was prolonged by 100% on each of the next two courses unless there was dose-limiting toxicity. The subsequent infusion durations were 48 and 96 hrs, and further prolongation of drug administration was not attempted. Peak plasma levels of total adriamycin fluorescence, which had been 1.3 micrograms/ml with standard rapid drug administration, decreased to 0.24, 0.13 and 0.10 micrograms/ml with 24-, 48-, and 96-hr infusions, respectively. Because of the risks of adriamycin extravasation, prolonged adriamycin infusions must be given with central-venous access. We have employed simple, percutaneous, silicone-elastomer, central-venous catheters and ambulatory infusion pumps for drug administration.

In the initial study, all patients had CMF-resistant breast cancer and were treated with single-agent adriamycin. We were concerned at the beginning of that study that therapeutic efficacy might be decreased; however, we obtained a 50% response rate and acceptable toxicity (21). As expected, the incidence of mucositis was somewhat higher than with rapid infusion. In contrast, nausea and vomiting were markedly decreased, especially with the longer infusion durations. We have subsequently studied continuous-infusion adriamycin administration in patients with sarcomas and breast cancer in front-line combination therapy without apparent loss of efficacy.

In a variety of studies we have utilized adriamycin infusions of different durations up to 96 hrs. The longer the infusion, the lower the peak drug level, the lower the cardiac toxicity. Table 3 shows the effects of infusion duration on the incidence of high-grade endomyocardial biopsies since that is the best measure of cardiac toxicity from the point of view of risk of developing CHF.

Table 3. High-Grade Endomyocardial Biopsies by Infusion Schedule

Cumulative Dose		Infusion Duration			
		Rapid	24 hr	48 hr	96 hr
401- 600	Number of Biopsies	28	15	27	42
	Percent High-grade	32	13	11	2
601- 800	Number of Biopsies	6	21	18	39
	Percent High-grade	33	24	11	5
801-1000	Number of Biopsies	0	6	5	36
	Percent High-grade	--	33	20	11
1001-1200	Number of Biopsies	0	0	0	21
	Percent High-grade	--	--	--	19
1201-1905	Number of Biopsies	0	0	0	9
	Percent High-grade	--	--	--	78

At each cumulative-dose level, the percent of patients with high-grade biopsies decreases with increasing infusion duration. Since these studies include only those patients who have received more than 500 mg/m^2 of adriamycin, many patients on the standard schedule were screened out prior to entry because of cardiac toxicity on a baseline biopsy at lower doses. The data, therefore, are weighted in favor of the standard infusion. Nonetheless, few patients treated with standard adriamycin were able to exceed a dose of 600 mg/m^2, and of those, one-third had high-grade biopsies. At doses of 800 to 1000 mg/m^2, one-third of patients with 24-hr adriamycin had high-grade biopsies as did 20% of those with 48-hr adriamycin. At 1000 to 1200 mg/m^2, about 20% of the patients with 96-hr adriamycin showed high-grade biopsies, and above 1200 mg/m^2, at doses up to 1900 mg/m^2, eventually 78% of the patients with 96-hr adriamycin showed high-grade cardiac biopsies.

We currently recommend that adriamycin be administered only by 48- to 96-hr continuous infusion. Cumulative doses of 600 mg/m^2 by 48-hr infusion and 800 mg/m^2 by 96-hr infusion can be given without additional cardiac monitoring and with less risk of producing CHF than with 450 mg/m^2 of standard adriamycin. For 96-hr adriamycin, we have treated over 50 patients to 800 mg/m^2 without causing CHF below that level (in the absence of other causes). Weekly adriamycin and 24-hr infusion, while clearly less cardiotoxic than standard adriamycin, do not offer a sufficient additional cumulative dose to be administered for potential therapeutic impact. We see no advantage for these schedules over the longer infusions unless the regimen causes dose-limiting mucositis.

A large number of anthracycline analogues have undergone preclinical trials and have been claimed to have decreased cardiac toxicity. Only two have had sufficient clinical evaluation for comment here, epirubicin and mitoxantrone. Jain demonstrated a statistically significant decrease in both CHF and decreased EF for epirubicin compared with adriamycin, even after correction for decreased potency (22). The magnitude of the advantage, however, is small, similar to that seen with weekly or 24-hr adriamycin infusion and less than that seen with 96-hr adriamycin (23). The intrinsic cardiac toxicity of epirubicin was substantially reduced by 48-hr continuous infusion (23).

Mitoxantrone is an anthraquinone lacking the amino-sugar of the true anthracyclines. Nonetheless, it does causes cardiac toxicity, morphologically identical to that of adriamycin and capable of producing CHF (24). After correction for differences in potency, mitoxantrone is substantially less cardiotoxic than adriamycin (25) and similar to 96-hr infusion adriamycin.

A number of free-radical scavengers have been used as cardio-protective agents with adriamycin. Myers first suggested that Vitamin E (alpha-tocopherol) could reduce lipid peroxidation caused by adriamycin in mouse myocardium (26). Similar effects were noted with N-acetylcysteine (27). Unfortunately, neither our trial with Vitamin E, utilizing cardiac biopsies (28), or Myers' trial with N-acetylcysteine, using EF's (29) demonstrated clinical cardio-protection.

Herman et al demonstrated cardioprotection with ICRF-187 but not with N-acetylcysteine in a chronic beagle-dog study (30). Preliminary data, reported this year by Green, confirm the cardioprotective effect in a clinical trial (31). These exciting results require further follow-up to determine the extent of the cardioprotection.

Conclusion

We have come a long way since the initial descriptions of adriamycin cardiomyopathy. Cumulative-dose limitation protects the majority of patients. Sophisticated cardiac monitoring with EF's and especially with cardiac biopsies permits quantitative study of new approaches to decrease the toxicity. Optimal scheduling with 96-hr infusions permits doubling of cumulative doses and still produces less cardiac toxicity. Newer less cardiotoxic analogues have been developed, and at least one drug, ICRF-187, has decreased adriamycin cardiac toxicity in a clinical trial. Anthracycline cardiac toxicity may become a problem of historical interest only.

REFERENCES

1. Lefrak, E.A., Pitha, J., Rosenheim, S., Gottlieb, J.A. (1973) Cancer 32: 302-314.

2. Minow, R.A., Benjamin, R.S., Lee, E.T., Gottlieb, J.A. (1977) Cancer 39: 1397-1402.

3. Von Hoff, D.D., Layard, M.W., Basas, P., et al. (1979) Ann Intern Med 91: 710-717.

4. Haq, M.M., Legha, S.S., Choksi, J., et al. (1985) Cancer 56: 1361-1365.

5. Billingham, M., Bristow, M.R., Glatstein, E., et al. (1977) Am J Surg Path 1: 17-23.

6. Bristow, M.R., Mason, J.W., Billingham, M.E., et al. (1978) Ann Intern Med 88: 169-175.

7. Mackay, B., Keyes, L.M., Benjamin, R.S., et al. (1981) TX Soc
    Electron Micro J 11: 7-15.

8. Legha, S.S., Benjamin, R.S., Mackay, B., et al. (1982) Ann
    Intern Med 96: 133-139.

9. Chawla, S.P., Benjamin, R.S., Legha, S.S., et al. (1983) IN:
    Proceedings of the 13th International Congress of Chemotherapy
    eds. Spitzy, K.H., and Karrer, K. (Verlag H. Egermann, Vienna),
    pp. 490-492.

10. Benjamin, R.S., Chawla, S.P., Hortobagyi, G.N., et al. (1986)
    IN: Clinical Applications of Continuous Infusion Chemotherapy
    and Concomitant Radiation Therapy eds. Rosenthal, C.J. and
    Rotman, M. (Plenum Press, New York), pp. 19-25.

11. Alexander, J., Dainiak, N., Berger, H.J., et al. (1979) NEJM
    300: 278-283.

12. Ewer, M.S., Ali, M.K., Chawla, S.P., et al. (1985) Proc Am Soc
    Clin Oncol 4: 27.

13. Blum, R.H., Carter, S.K. (1974) Ann Intern Med 80: 249-259.

14. Benjamin, R.S. (1975) Cancer Chemotherap Rep 6: 191-194.

15. Benjamin, R.S, Riggs C.E. Jr., and Bachur, N.R. (1973) Clinical
    Pharm and Therap 14: 592-600.

16. Benjamin, R.S., Wiernik, P.H., and Bachur, N.R. (1974) Cancer
    33: 19-37.

17. Weiss, A.J., Metter, G.E., Fletcher, W.S., et al. (1976) Cancer
    Treat Rep 60: 813-822.

18. Chlebowski, R.T., Paroly, W.S., Pugh, R.P., et al. (1980)
    Cancer Treat Rep 64: 47-51.

19. Valdivieso, M., Burgess, M.A., Ewer, M.S., et al. (1984) J Clin
    Oncology 2: 207-214.

20. Torti, F.M., Bristow, M.R., Howes, A.E., et al. (1983) Ann
    Intern Med 99: 745-749.

21. Legha, S.S., Benjamin, R.S., Mackay, B, et al. (1982) Cancer
    49: 1763-1766.

22. Jain, K.K., Casper, E. S. Geller, N.L., et al. (1985) J Clin
    Oncol 3: 818-826.

23. Chawla, S.P., Benjamin, R.S., Hortobagyi, G.N. et al. (1986)
    Proc Am Soc Clin Oncol 5: 44.

24. Benjamin, R.S., Holmes, F, Chawla, S.P., et al. (1985) Current
    Status of Navatrone pp 69-73.

25. Dukart, G., Posner, L., Henry, D., et al. (1986) Proc Am Soc
    Clin Oncol 5: 48.

26. Myers, C.E, McGuire, W.P. Liss, R.H, et al. (1977) Science 197:
    165-167.

27. Doroshow, J.H., Locker, G.Y, Ifrim, I., et al. (1981) J Clin
    Invest 64: 1053-1056.

28. Legha, S.S, Wang, Y.M., Mackay, B, et al. (1982) Ann NY Acad
    Sci 393: 411-418.

29. Myers, C., Bonow, R., Palmeri, S., et al. (1983) Sem Oncol 10:
    53-55.

30. Herman, E.H., Ferrans, V.J., Myers, C.E., and Van Vleet, J.F.
    (1985) Cancer Research 45: 276-381

31. Green, M.D., Speyer, J.L., Stecy, P., et al. (1987) Proc Am Soc
    Clin Oncol 6: 28.

Pretreatment with ICRF-187 Protects Against the Chronic Cardiac Toxicity Produced by Very Large Cumulative Doses of Doxorubicin in Beagle Dogs
V.J. Ferrans, E.H. Herman, and R.L. Hamlin

The optimal use of anthracyclines, such as doxorubicin and daunorubicin, in cancer chemotherapy is hampered by the serious cardiotoxicity that these agents produce when administered to patients. This cardiac toxicity can be acute, subacute and chronic. The acute cardiotoxicity is manifested immediately after the drug is given and consists of hypotension and electrocardiographic changes, which have been attributed to acute, drug-induced release of histamine. The subacute toxicity is rare and is clinically evident in the form of transient myocarditis and pericarditis. The chronic toxicity is the most important and consists of dilated cardiomyopathy, which may have a delayed onset, is often fatal, and usually occurs when the drug is given in cumulative doses which exceed 450 mg/m^2 (1).

Numerous efforts have been made to decrease or eliminate the chronic cardiotoxicity of anthracyclines without compromising their antineoplastic effects. Among these efforts are: 1) modified dose scheduling, in which the anthracyclines are administered by very slow (96 hours) intravenous infusions instead of bolus injections; 2) development of less cardiotoxic analogues, such as 4'epidoxorubicin; 3) use of modified drug delivery systems, such as encapsulation of the drug into liposomes or complexing with other substances such as dextran or DNA, and 4) the administration of agents which would protect the myocardium from anthracycline toxicity. The latter agents include: cysteamine, N-acetylcysteine, vitamin E, ubiquinone and ICRF-187. The use of most of these agents is based upon the premises that 1) the cardiotoxic effects of anthracyclines are consequences of the formation of cytotoxic oxygen free radicals which produce myocyte damage and 2) that these compounds can scavenge free radicals (1). The most successful cardiac protective agent is ICRF-187, which is not a free radical scavenger, but which appears to function by chelating iron ions that are needed for the anthracycline-mediated formation of free radicals (2).

ICRF-187, (+)-1,2-bis(3,5-dioxoketopiperazin-1-yl)propane, a derivative of ethylenediaminetetraacetic acid, is the more soluble d-isomer of ICRF-159, the compound that originally was studied by Creighton et al. (3) and found to exert some antineoplastic activity and to enhance, rather than to interfere with, the antitumor activity of daunorubicin (4, 5). ICRF-187 and ICRF-159 significantly reduce the lethal effects of high doses of daunorubicin in Syrian golden hamsters (6, 7) and in mice (8). In additional experiments, Herman et al. (9) showed that the severity of the toxicity produced by a single (25 mg/kg) dose of daunorubicin was reduced by pretreatment with ICRF-187 at doses of 12.5 mg/kg or greater. Although most animals pretreated with 12.5 to 50 mg/kg of ICRF-187 were alive after 5 weeks, their body weights were below control levels. Animals pretreated with 100 mg/kg of ICRF-187 were the only group able to regain initial weight loss and to increase body weight above the initial preinjection level. Different degrees of protection were observed when the 100 mg/kg dose of ICRF-187 was given at various times before and after the dose of daunorubicin. Significant numbers of animals (45%) survived when ICRF-187 was given 48 hours before daunorubicin; however, survival was optimal when ICRF-187 was given from 3 hours before to 3 hours after daunorubicin, and the protective effect was lost when ICRF-187 was administered more than 6 hours after daunorubicin. Histopathologic observations suggest: 1) that under the conditions of this study, alterations in heart, liver or kidneys did not appear to be of sufficient magnitude to be responsible for the lethality in the hamsters and 2) that the lethal effects of a single, high dose of daunorubicin are due to profound gastrointestinal toxicity, and that this toxicity is altered by ICRF-187.

We have made detailed comparisons of the protective activity of
ICRF-187 and a series of structurally related bis-dioxopiperazine
analogues against acute daunorubicin toxicity in Syrian golden hamsters (10). A single dose of 25 mg/kg of daunorubicin was lethal to
84% of the animals within 1 to 4 weeks. Over 70% of animals given
50 to 200 mg/kg of ICRF-187 before daunorubicin were alive at 8
weeks. Similar results were obtained with ICRF-186, the l-isomer of
ICRF-159, indicating that the protective activity is not stereospeci-
fic. Eighteen other analogues were evaluated for prospective activity; only bimolane, a central chain desmethyl analogue of ICRF-187
with N-morpholinomethyl substituents in each dioxopiperazine ring,
was as effective as ICRF-187 in reducing the mortality of daunorubicin. The role of the N-morpholinomethyl groups in the biological
activity of bimolane needs further study since ICRF-154, a similar
compound without these substituents, exerted only minimal protective
activity. Protection against daunorubicin lethality was minimal or
absent when hamsters were pretreated with various doses of ICRF-187
analogues in which slight changes had been made in the dioxopiperazine rings (ICRF-158, ICRF-198) or in the central chain (ICRF-161,
ICRF-192, ICRF-193, ICRF-197, ICRF-198 and ICRF-202). Similarly,
animals treated with a number of conformationally constrained cyclo-
propane analogues of bis-dioxopiperazine compounds before receiving
daunorubicin died at the same rates as those given only daunorubicin.
These results indicate that very little alteration can occur in the
basic structure of ICRF-187 without loss of its protective activity.
In other studies it has been found that ICRF-187 (or the acid hydrolysis product of its ring structures) has a high affinity for iron
and other divalent cations (11), and that this compound protects
against two other types of toxicity in which cell damage is produced
through the iron-catalyzed formation of free radicals, namely,
acetaminophen-induced liver damage (12) and alloxan-induced damage
to pancreatic beta cells with resulting diabetes mellitus (13). The
effects of analogues of ICRF-187 on these toxicities have not been
studied yet. It remains to be determined whether chelation of divalent ions differentiates compounds with high cardioprotective activity (ICRF-187, ICRF-186 and bimolane) from those having little or no

cardioprotection.

A series of investigations has demonstrated that ICRF-159 and ICRF-187 are effective in blocking the chronic cardiotoxicity produced by doxorubicin in experimental animals treated with doses of this agent which are similar to those employed in clinical medicine in the cancer chemotherapy of human patients. These beneficial effects have been noted in beagle dogs (14-16), miniature swine (15, 17), rabbits (15, 18), spontaneously hypertensive rats (SHR), and normotensive Wistar-Kyoto rats (WKY), which are the strain most closely related genetically to the SHR (19). For reasons that are not clear at present, SHR are considerably more sensitive than WKY to the cardiotoxic effects of doxorubicin; however, they show the usual cardioprotective response to the administration of ICRF-187 with doxorubicin (19). In rabbits (20), we were able to demonstrate that the cardioprotection produced by ICRF-187 is long-lasting. Rabbits were given 3.2 mg/kg of daunorubicin, with or without pretreatment with 25 mg/kg of ICRF-187, once every 3 weeks over an 18-week period (6 doses). The experiment was terminated 3 months after the last treatment. At this time, all 7 rabbits given daunorubicin alone has evidence of myocardial alterations ranging from minimal (2 animals) to mild (5 animals). Pretreatment with ICRF-187 caused a significant reduction in both the incidence and the severity of the cardiac lesions: hearts from 5 to 7 animals given the combination of ICRF-187 and daunorubicin were normal, and alterations were minimal in the other 2 animals. Thus, this study demonstrates that pretreatment with ICRF-187 provides prolonged protection against the cardiomyopathy, as opposed to producing only a delay in the appearance of the cardiac alterations. Another study, in beagle dogs, confirmed the effectiveness of ICRF-187 in reducing the severity of doxorubicin-induced cardiomyopathy, and also showed that the concurrent administration of N-acetylcysteine did not improve the effectiveness of ICRF-187, and that by itself, N-acetylcysteine did not provide significant protection in the context of the chronic cardiomyopathy induced by doxorubicin (16).

All the studies mentioned above had been carried out with the usual therapeutic doses of anthracyclines, and the important question

of whether or not higher doses of anthracyclines would be tolerated
by animals pretreated with ICRF-187 had not been addressed. Therefore, another study was initiated to examine the influence of ICRF-
187 on functional and morphological aspects of the cardiotoxicity
produced by high doses of doxorubicin over a prolonged period of
time. In this study, 27 beagle dogs were subdivided into 4 groups.
Groups 1 and 2 (n = 8) received 1.75 mg/kg of doxorubicin intravenously at 3 week intervals; animals in group 2 were pretreated with
25 mg/kg of ICRF-187 intravenously. Dogs in group 3 (n = 5) received
ICRF-187 alone, and those in group 4 (n = 5) received saline alone.
Animals in all groups were subjected to a number of studies, including: measurements of systolic, diastolic and mean arterial blood
pressure; electrocardiograms; echocardiograms; hematological evaluations, and blood or serum determinations of urea nitrogen, creatinine, glucose, total proteins, albumin, globulin, direct and total
bilirubin, total lipids, triglycerides, uric acid, sodium, potassium,
calcium, chloride, phosphorus, glutamic-pyruvic transaminase, gluta-
mic-oxaloacetic transaminase, lactic dehydrogenase and creatine
kinase. These studies were made two times before the beginning of
drug administration and were repeated at three-week intervals thereafter until termination of the study. Two-tailed paired sample
statistical analysis was performed to evaluate the significance of
treatment-related differences in the results obtained.

At the time of spontaneously occurring death or terminal elec-
tive study, necropsies were performed and samples of tissues from
all major organs were fixed in formalin and examined histologically.
The frequency and severity of doxorubicin-induced cardiac lesions
were evaluated by light microscopic examination of left ventricular
tissue. The changes observed were graded on a scale of 0 to 4+ on
the basis of the numbers of msucle cells showing cytoplasmic vacuolization and myofibrillar loss, in which 0 = no lesions; 1+ = involvement of only an occasional cell; 4+ = involvement of 50% or
more of the cells, and 2+ and 3+ = intermediate degrees of involvement. Differences in the severity scores of the groups were evaluated using the chi square test. A lesions score of 2+ was arbitra-
rily chosen as the level for determining whether or not significant

protective effects were being obtained.

Five of the eight dogs given doxorubicin alone died during the
course of the study: 2 died after receiving 7 doses (12.25 mg/kg) and
3 died after 8 doses (14 mg/kg). The remaining 3 animals in this
group were euthanatized while in poor condition after 8 doses. Four
of 8 dogs given doxorubicin and ICRF-187 died during the study: 1
died after the 20th dose (35 mg/kg); 2 after the 25th dose (43.75
mg/kg) and 1 after the 30th dose (42.5 mg/kg). Two other animals
were euthanatized after 25 injections (43.75 mg/kg) because of difficulty in continuing intravenous dosing, and 2 animals survived all 30
dosings (52.5 mg/kg). None of the animals given ICRF-187 alone or
saline died during the study. Alopecia was observed in dogs receiving doxorubicin, beginning after the third dose; ICRF-187 did not
protect against this change.

Electrocardiographic changes observed in the dogs receiving
doxorubicin alone consisted mainly of ventricular premature beats.
In the dogs receiving doxorubicin plus ICRF-187, changes developed
only after 15 doses (i.e., approximately 300 days) and consisted of
prolongation of the PQ interval. Occasionally this progressed to
2nd or 3rd degree AV block. By 425 days, other changes were observed
which consisted of widening, decrease in amplitude and development
of high frequency components in the QRS. Finally, by 550 days, ventricular premature beats were frequently present. Echocardiograms
and measurements of arterial pressure did not show important differences between the different groups of animals. Similarly, clinical
laboratory studies did not show important treatment-related differences between the various groups.

Alterations in the liver (hepatic congestion), kidney (congestion) and small intestine (loss of epithelial cells at the tips of
the villi and associated inflammatory cell reaction) were found in
dogs receiving doxorubicin alone. These changes were very infre-
quent in the dogs receiving doxorubicin and ICRF-187 and were absent
in the other 2 groups of dogs. The most frequent change observed in
dogs given the combination of doxorubicin and ICRF-187 was a marked
decrease in lymphoid tissue. Testicular atrophy was evident in the
2 dogs that had tolerated 30 injections of doxorubicin and ICRF-187.

No consistent abnormalities were found in the tissues from animals that had received up to 30 doses of ICRF-187 alone or saline.

On histologic study, myocardial lesions of marked degree (3+) were observed in each of the 8 animals given doxorubicin alone (12.25 to 14 mg/kg). In contrast, dogs pretreated with ICRF-187 received much higher doses of doxorubicin (35 to 52.5 mg/kg) and showed significant decreases in the incidence and severity of cardiac lesions. No cardiac lesions were found in 4 of 5 dogs pretreated with ICRF-187 and given cumulative doses of 35 to 43.75 mg/kg of doxorubicin. The severity of the lesions in the remaining 4 dogs pretreated with ICRF-187 was 1+ in 2 animals given 43.75 and 52.5 mg/kg of doxorubicin, respectively, and 2+ in 2 animals given 52.5 mg/kg of doxorubicin. No cardiac lesions were present in dogs receiving ICRF-187 or saline alone.

The results summarized above indicate clearly that pretreatment with ICRF-187 makes it possible to administer much higher cumulative doses of doxorubicin than are tolerable without this pretreatment. In fact, such doses of doxorubicin as we have been able to give, together with ICRF-187, to beagle dogs (up to 52.5 mg/kg) are greatly in excess of those (12-16 mg/kg) which produce severe cardiomyopathy when given without ICRF-187. Thus, these results confirm and extend our previous observations concerning the effectiveness of ICRF-187 against doxorubicin-induced cardiomyopathy. They also suggest that doxorubicin may be used together with ICRF-187 in the clinical practice of Oncology and that the consequent elimination of cardiotoxicity will make it possible to administer much higher doses of doxorubicin to human patients than is possible at the present time.

REFERENCES

1. Myers, C.E. (1987) Proc. Organ Directed Toxicities of Anticancer Drugs, First International Symposium. Burlington, VT, June 4-6, p. 5.
2. Myers, C.E., Gianni, L., Simone, C.B., Klecker, R., and Greene R. (1982) Biochemistry 21: 1707-1713.
3. Creighton, A.M., Hellman, K. and Whitecross S. (1969) Nature 222: 384-385.
4. Woodman, R.J., Cysyk, R.C., Kline, I., Gang, M. and Venditti, J.M. (1975) Cancer Chemother. Rep. 59: 689-695.
5. Giuliani, F., Casazza, A.M., Di Marco, A. and Savi, G. (1981) Cancer Treat. Rep. 65: 267-276.

6. Herman, E.H., Mhatre, R.M. and Chadwick, DP. (1974) Toxicol. Appl. Pharmacol. 27: 517-526.

7. Herman, E.H., Ardalan, B., Bier, C., Warakdevar, V. and Krop, S. (1979) Cancer Treat. Rep. 63: 89-92.

8. Wang, G., Finch, M.D., Trevan, D. and Hellman, K. (1981) Br. J. Cancer 43: 871-877.

9. Herman, E.H., El-Hage, A.N., Ferrans, V.J. and Witiak, D.T. (1983) Res. Commun. Chem. Pathol. Pharmacol. 40: 217-231.

10. Herman, E.H., El-Hage, A.N., Creighton, A.M., Witiak, D.T. and Ferrans, V.J. (1985) Res. Commun. Chem. Pathol. Pharmacol. 48: 39-55.

11. El-Hage, A.N., Herman, E.H., Yang, G.C., Crouch, R.K. and Ferrans, V.J. (1986) Res. Commun. Chem. Pathol. Pharmacol. 52: 341-360.

12. El-Hage, A.N., Herman, E.H. and Ferrans, V.J. (1983) Toxicology 28: 295-303.

13. El-Hage, A.N., Herman, E.H. and Ferrans, V.J. (1981) Res. Commun. Chem. Pathol. Pharmacol. 33: 509-523.

14. Herman, E.H. and Ferrans, V.J. (1981) Cancer Res. 41: 3436-3440.

15. Herman, E.H. and Ferrans, V.J. (1983) Drugs Exp. Clin. Res. 9: 483-490.

16. Herman, E.H., Ferrans, V.J., Myers, C.E. and Van Vleet, J.F. (1985) Cancer 45: 276-281.

17. Herman, E.H. and Ferrans, V.J. (1983) Lab. Invest. 49: 69-77.

18. Herman, E.H., Ferrans, V.J., Jordan, W. and Ardalan, B. (1981) Res. Commun. Chem. Pathol. Pharmacol. 31: 85-97.

19. Herman, E.H., El-Hage, A.N., Ferrans, V.J. and Ardalan, B. (1985) Toxicol. Appl. Pharmacol. 78: 202-214.

20. Herman, E.H. and Ferrans, V.J. (1986) Cancer Chemother. Pharmacol. 16: 102-106.

A Trial of ICRF-187 to Selectively Protect Against Chronic Adriamycin Cardiac Toxicity: Rationale and Preliminary Results of a Clinical Trial

J.L. Speyer, M.D. Green, C. Ward, J. Sanger, E. Kramer, M. Rey, J.C. Wernz, R.H. Blum, M. Meyers, F.M. Muggia, V. Ferrans, P. Stecy, F. Feit, N. Dubin, A. Jacquotte, S. Taubes, and C. London

The wide spectrum of anthracycline activity as well as the unique cumulative dose related cardiac toxicity pose a significant clinical challenge. These drugs, particularly doxorubicin (Adriamycin^R), constitute some of the most active compounds available to the clinical oncologist. They have activity in both hematologic malignancies and solid tumors. Numerous efforts to improve upon their activity through analogue development or a better dose schedule of administration have not substantially altered the anti-tumor activity. Further efforts in this area may yet bear fruit. However, at the present time the challenge to improve the therapeutic ratio must be met by reducing toxicity, particularly cardiac toxicity.

Reduction in anthracycline-induced cardiac toxicity is relevant not only to situations where responding patients might receive Adriamycin beyond the conventional cumulative stopping dose level of 450 mg/m^2 - 550 mg/m^2, but to a large group of patients who never receive Adriamycin because of perceived risk of cardiac toxicity. This group includes patients who may have increased risk with standard doses because they have one or more of the conventionally identified risk factors (age greater than 65, preexisting myocardial muscle dysfunction or prior chest wall radiation) (1). Perhaps even more important in this group are those patients receiving adjuvant chemotherapy, in whom even a modest risk of developing cardiomyopathy may unacceptably offset the possible benefits of therapy.

Analogue development has some promise but has not yet provided a major breakthrough in clinical practice. 4'Epidoxorubicin, deoxy-doxorubicin and mitoxantrone are currently in use in Europe but reports of decreased cardiac toxicity are inconclusive or conflicting and antitumor efficacy is not always maintained.

Changes in dose and schedule have provided important benefits, though not without additional costs. Pharmacokinetic data suggest that peak plasma levels rather than total area under the curve may be related to cardiac toxicity. This has led to testing of continuous infusion schedules of Adriamycin. As reviewed by Dr. Benjamin elsewhere in this volume, studies at the MD Anderson and in other institutions (2, 3) with infusion schedules up to 96 hours in duration have yielded decreased cardiac toxicity as measured by cardiac exam, nuclear gated pool scan and endomyocardial biopsy. However, the desirability of this approach is limited by the need for indwelling catheters with external pumps as well as an increased and perhaps dose limiting mucositis.

Agents which may selectively block the development of cardiac toxicity without interfering with antitumor activity have been investigated. The rationale for this approach assumes that cardiac toxicity and antitumor effect occur either by separate mechanisms or that the "protective" agent selectively rescues normal cells and not tumor cells. Germinal studies in mice by Myers et al (4) suggested that Adriamycin-induced cardiac toxicity could be blocked by the free radical scavenger alpha tocopherol without interfering with antitumor activity.

Elegant studies reviewed in this volume by Drs. Myers (5) and Doroshow (6) have shed considerable light on the mechanism of anthracycline-induced cardiac toxicity. These authors demonstrated that 1) Adriamycin undergoes chemical or enzymatic conversions which generate free radical $\cdot OH$ and H_2O_2, 2) at least one pathway of these interconversions requires the reduction of Fe^{3+} to Fe^{2+} in an Adriamycin-Fe complex, 3) mechanisms exist in cardiac cells to facilitate the generation of oxyradicals, 4) these oxyradicals can directly damage myocytes at several intracellular locations, 5) this intracellular site specific damage may depend on the availability of utilizable iron i.e. in ferritin and 6) mammalian cardiac cells, in fact, have poor enzymatic defenses against this kind of oxyradical damage when compared to cells from other organs. The search for appropriate and selective blocking agents has focused on interdicting these free radical mechanisms. However, early clinical trials with alpha tocopherol, superoxide dismutase and N-acetyl cysteine have not yet been successful.

An independent line of research has led us to test ICRF-187 as a cardioprotective agent. This compound (see structure) is a bisdioxopiperazine. It was originally synthesized by Dr. Andrew Creighton of the Imperial Cancer Research Fund (ICRF) as a possible anticancer drug. It is an analogue of EDTA which appears to undergo acid hydrolysis of the ring structures to form a bidentate chelator which has high affinity for iron, copper and other metals. Dr. Eugene Herman of the U.S. FDA tested ICRF-159 (ICRF-187 is the enantiomer of this compound) in an isolated heart-lung preparation and observed that it inhibited Adriamycin-induced increases in coronary perfusion pressure (7). In a series of extensive experiments by Drs. Herman and Ferrans (see Chapter by Dr. Ferrans in this volume) (8), it was demonstrated that ICRF-159 (9) or its more soluble form ICRF-187 could block chronic Adriamycin-induced cardiac toxicity in mice, rats, Syrian golden hamsters, miniature swine, rabbits and beagle dogs (10). In their experiments and those of others, cardiac protection did not extend to other toxicities. It did not protect against alopecia or bone marrow suppression and was variable in preventing mucositis. More important, ICRF-187 did not block the antitumor effect of doxorubicin against L1210 leukemia. Further support to test this compound comes from the fact that it blocks known free radical dependent biologic processes such as acetaminophen hepatotoxicity and experimental Alloxan-induced diabetes.

Based upon this preclinical data, it appeared reasonable to test ICRF-187 in the setting of potential Adriamycin-induced cardiac toxicity. Phase I (11) and II clinical trials of ICRF-187 (11) demonstrated that myelosuppression is the dose limiting toxicity, at a dose level of 1500 mg/m^2 x 3 days q 3 weeks. Scaling up from the animal data, cardioprotection occurs in the range of 1:10 to 1:15 ratio of Adriamycin to ICRF-187 by weight. Recent confirmatory studies (12) using the Bertazzoli mouse model have confirmed this relationship. It can therefore be expected that a cardiac sparing dose of ICRF-187 should be considerably lower than doses required to cause systemic toxicity.

ICRF-187

ICRF-159 = - enantiomer

At New York University Medical Center we are conducting a randomized trial to determine if ICRF-187 can prevent cumulative Adriamycin-induced cardiac toxicity. Women receiving first-line chemotherapy for metastatic breast cancer are eligible for the study. This patient group was selected because it provided a relatively uniform group who would receive a single standard Adriamycin-containing regimen. Adriamycin is an active drug in this disease with a high response rate and prolonged duration of response. It would be expected that a significant number of these breast cancer patients would reach cumulative doses of drug at levels high enough to place them at risk for cardiac toxicity. Because these patients have advanced lesions, it is not unreasonable to continue treatment for persistent disease beyond this cumulative dose level provided that patients are closely monitored for deterioration in cardiac function. It is precisely this patient population that would enable us to adequately evaluate the cardioprotective effect of ICRF-187. The lower response rate of Adriamycin in other solid tumors or the practice of limited chemotherapy in the adjuvant setting would not make these situations suitable to this type of investigation. Our prior cardiac monitoring studies in this group of patients (13) has confirmed the acceptability of this model.

Eligibility criteria are shown in Table I. Patients have received no prior anthracycline therapy, are free of active cardiac disease and have a resting left ventricular ejection fraction (LVEF) as measured by gated radionucleotide scan of $\leq$ 0.45. Prior to randomization (Fig I) patients are stratified for prior adjuvant chemotherapy and cardiac risk factors (age greater than 65, prior cardiac disease, and chest wall radiation).

Table I
ELIGIBILITY CRITERIA

Histologic proof of breast cancer
Advanced disease
No prior anthracyclines
Adjuvant CMF > 6 mos prior to entry
ECOG PS 0-3
Informed consent
Bone marrow
   > 4000 WBC
   > 100,000 Platelets
Hepatic function
   < 3.0 Bilirubin
Cardiac function
   No active heart disease
   > 0.45 LVEF

Figure I
STRATIFICATION FACTORS

1. Cardiac risk
2. Prior adjuvant therapy

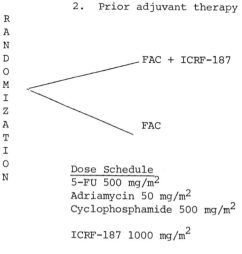

R
A
N
D
O
M
I
Z
A
T
I
O
N

FAC + ICRF-187

FAC

Dose Schedule
5-FU 500 mg/m^2
Adriamycin 50 mg/m^2
Cyclophosphamide 500 mg/m^2

ICRF-187 1000 mg/m^2

IV q 21 days

All patients are treated every three weeks with a standard chemotherapy regimen of 5-Fluorouracil 500 mg/m^2, Adriamycin 50 mg/m^2 (5-10 minute infusion) and Cyclophosphamide 500 mg/m^2 (FAC). Patients randomized to ICRF-187 receive 1000 mg/m^2 as an intravenous infusion 30 minutes prior to Adriamycin. Standard dose reduction criteria are followed. However, in order to prevent possible additive myelosuppression from ICRF-187 and its biasing the trial by reducing the Adriamycin dose, reductions in doses of chemotherapy during the first two cycles are made only in the doses of 5-FU and cyclophosphamide and not of Adriamycin.

Cardiac monitoring is threefold. It involves a clinical evaluation of the patient with physical examination, resting pulse rate, EKG, CXR (cardiothoracic ratio) and NY Heart Association Classification. Physiologic measure of myocardial contractibility is assessed by resting nuclear gated pool scans. These scans are performed prior to treatment and at pre-established cumulative doses of Adriamycin (300 mg/m^2, 450 mg/m^2 and each 100 mg/m^2 thereafter). Scans are performed 2 and 3 weeks after the last dose of Adriamycin. When possible, concurrent exercise scans are also performed. Finally all patients are offered endomyocardial biopsy at a cumulative dose level of 450 mg/m^2 of Adriamycin. All histopathology specimens are reviewed by one pathologist, Dr. Ferrans of the NHLBI.

All evaluations by the cardiologists, nuclear medicine physicians and pathologist were performed without prior knowledge of whether the patients were receiving ICRF-187. Endpoints of the study are either disease progression or cardiac toxicity. Patients are not removed from study at a predetermined cumulative dose of Adriamycin. Cardiac criteria for removal include: 1) development of clinical congestive heart failure, 2) a fall in LVEF to less than 0.45 or a fall from baseline LVEF by greater than 0.20, and 3) an endomyocardial biopsy score of $\geq$ 2.0 (Billingham system) (14).

The study is currently accruing patients and results are preliminary. Eighty two patients have been randomized with 41 patients in each arm. Treatment groups are balanced in terms of age, performance status, prior adjuvant chemotherapy, hormonal therapy, radiation therapy, and cardiac risk factors.

At this point in time, if we examine only patients who are off study, the amount of treatment is similar: FAC - mean number of cycles 8.5, mean cumulative Adriamycin dose 394 mg/m^2 and FAC + ICRF-187 - mean number of cycles 9.7, mean cumulative Adriamycin dose 474 mg/m^2. These differences are not statistically significant.

At this time only one patient on the FAC arm has received greater than 600 mg/m^2 while 9 patients on the FAC + ICRF-187 arm have received greater than 600 mg/m^2 of Adriamycin with 3 patients receiving 1000 mg/m^2. This difference does not appear to be due to differences in progression, tumor response, or non-cardiac toxicities, but rather to fewer patients on the FAC + ICRF-187 arm being removed from study for cardiac toxicity. Forty two percent of patients on FAC vs 45% of patients on FAC + ICRF-187 were removed for disease progression. Objective response rates in both arms are balanced at FAC - 46% and FAC + ICRF-187 - 47%, with CRs and PRs also being balanced. There is also no difference in the median time to disease progressions 9.2 months FAC vs 10.1 months FAC + ICRF-187. Non-cardiac toxicities are also similar in both arms of the study (15). The treatment groups are balanced for hematologic suppression, infections, fever and neutropenia, treatment deaths, alopecia and mucositis. Patients in the FAC vs FAC + ICRF-187 arm have received 90% vs 95% respectively of the predicted dose of Adriamycin and 85% vs 83.5% respectively of the predicted dose of Cytoxan and 5-FU.

Cardiac protection is suggested by these results. The conclusion is preliminary and cannot be stated with certainty at this time as the study is still open to accrual. Nine patients in the FAC arm and 2 patients in the FAC + ICRF-187 arm have developed clinical cardiac failure. The resting LVEF demonstrates protection by ICRF-187. Protection against Adriamycin-induced falls in LVEF occur even at relatively low dose ranges. The mean fall from baseline LVEF in patients with a cumulative Adriamycin dose of 300-395 mg/m^2 is 6.6 for the FAC patients and 1.6 for the FAC plus ICRF patients, $p < .04$. This difference persists at the higher dose levels of 500-599 mg/m^2 where the mean fall in LVEF is 15.8 for the FAC patients vs 2.1 for the FAC + ICRF-187, $p < .001$. However, because of the small number of patients at the higher dose levels, the power of the observation in patients receiving greater than 500 mg/m^2 is not sufficiently great to be conclusive.

The results of endomyocardial biopsies are not currently available and will be presented along with more complete data and the entire group of patients in a subsequent publication.

If these results are confirmed, not only by additional information from this study but by other studies as well, it will document the first time that we have been able to selectively block chronic Adriamycin-induced cardiomyopathy without interfering with antitumor activity of the drug. This protection appears to occur at doses of ICRF-187 which do not add to the non-cardiac toxicity of the FAC regimen. It is possible that somehow the FAC drug regimen or patients with breast cancer are unique. Confirmatory studies will need to examine the combination of ICRF-187 and Adriamycin in both the setting of other malignancies and other drug combinations before we can accept this selective cardioprotection as a generalized phenomenon.

If it is confirmed, these observations can provide important leads to further probe the mechanism of anthracycline-induced cardiac and non-cardiac damage. The role of iron or of ICRF-187 as an iron chelator has not been completely established. Morphologic studies of ferritin content in the cardiac biopsies from this study are being conducted by Dr. Luc Gianni - NCI Milan.

Recent observations by Doroshow (16, 17) and Sinha (18) indicate that free radical generation may be important not only in myocardial toxicity, but in the antitumor activity of Adriamycin. While this needs to be confirmed, and the relative role of this effect vis a vis DNA intercalating mechanisms determined, it raises an interesting set of questions relating to ICRF-187. If Adriamycin generates a variety of iron requiring oxyradical mediated sites of activity and damage, then ICRF-187 might be expected to block all of them. The differences in the protective effects of ICRF-187 between myocardial or other systemic sites and tumor cells (since antitumor effect was not decreased in our trial or in preclinical systems) may lie in the bioavailability of active drug in host cells and tumor cells. Clearly, this is conjecture at this time.

Finally if ICRF-187 does block oxyradical induced anthracycline injury then it may be useful to examine this drug in other clinical settings where free radical production appears to have a role. Bleomycin pulmonary toxicity with a known iron requirement and reoxygenation injury after coronary occlusion or bypass are both worthy of consideration.

ACKNOWLEDGEMENTS

Supported in part by CA 36524, CA 16087, CRC 96 and the Lila Motley Fund. The authors wish to acknowledge the many physicians and nurses who participated in the care of the patients and as well as the patients who consented to participate in this trial. We also wish to acknowledge Ms. Peggy Nixdorf for assistance in manuscript preparation.

REFERENCES

1. Von Hoff, D.D., Layard, M.W., Basa, P., et al. (1979) Ann. Intern. Med. 91: 710-717.
2. Benjamin, R.S., Chawla, S.P., Ewer, M.S., Hortobagyi, G.N., Mackay, B., Legha, S.S., Carrasco, C.H., Wallace, S. (1987) Proc. Organ Directed Toxicities of Anticancer Drugs, First International Symposium. Burlington, VT, June 4-6, p. 9.
3. Legha, S.S., Benjamin, R.S., Mackay, B., et al. (1982) Ann. Intern. Med. 96: 133-139.
4. Myers, C.E., McGuire, W.P., Liss, R.H., et al. (1977) Science. 197: 165-167.
5. Myers, C.E. (1987) Proc. Organ Directed Toxicities of Anticancer Drugs, First International Symposium. Burlington, VT, June 4-6, p. 5.
6. Doroshow, J.H. (1987) Proc. Organ Directed Toxicities of Anticancer Drugs, First International Symposium. Burlington, VT, June 4-6, p. 7.
7. Herman, E.H., Mhatre, R.M., Lee, I.P., and Waravdekar, V.S. (1972) Proc. Soc. Exp. Biol. Med. 140: 234-239.
8. Ferrans, V.J., Herman, E.H., and Hamlin, R.L. (1987) Proc. Organ Directed Toxicities of Anticancer Drugs, First International Symposium. Burlington, VT, June 4-6, p. 11.
9. Herman, E., Mhatre, R, and Chadwick, D. (1974) Toxicol. Appl. Pharmacol. 27: 517-527.
10. Herman, E.H., Ferrans, V.J. (1981) Cancer Res. 41: 3436-3440.
11. Von Hoff, D.D., Howser, D., Lewis, B.J., et al. (1981) Cancer Treat Rep. 65: 249-252.
12. Filppi, J.A., Imondi, A.R., Wolgemuth, R.L. (1987) Proc. Organ Directed Toxicities of Anticancer Drugs, First International Symposium. Burlington, VT, June 4-6, p. 22.

13. Speyer, J.L., Green, M.D., Dubin, N., Blum, R.H., Wernz, J.C., Roses, D., Sanger, J., and Muggia, F.M. (1985) Am. J. Med. 78: 555-563.

14. Bristow, M.R., Mason, J.W., Billingham, M.E., Daniels, J.R. (1981) Amer. Heart J. 102: 709-718.

15. Green, M.D., Speyer, J.L., Stecy, P., Rey, M., Kramer, E., Sanger, J., Feit, F., Blum, R.H., Wernz, J.C., Ward, C., London, C., Dubin, N., Muggia, F.M. (1987) Proc. Am. Soc. Clin. Onc. 104, p. 28.

16. Doroshow, J.H. (1986) Biochem. Biophys. Res. Commun. 135: 330-335.

17. Doroshow, J.H. (1986) Proc. Natl. Acad. Sci. (USA). 83: 4514-4518.

18. Sinha, B., Katki, A., Batist, G., Cowan, K., and Myers, C. (In Press) Biochemistry.

SECTION II

BLEOMYCIN INDUCED PULMONARY TOXICITY

Chaired by J.S. Lazo

Overview
J.S. Lazo

Pulmonary injury is a frequent untoward effect of antineoplastic therapy. Of particular concern is pulmonary fibrosis, a potentially lethal response of the lungs to not only antineoplastic agents but also to a host of other drugs and environmental substances. Pulmonary fibrosis is the most serious untoward effect of the bleomycins. Many research laboratories have used the bleomycins as experimental tools to uncover the basic mechanisms in the pathogenesis of pulmonary fibrosis, to identify early means of detection, and to discover new pharmacologic approaches to mitigate fibrosis. The goal of the following chapters was to outline recent advances in these areas.

The chemical interactions between the bleomycins and their presumed target, DNA, were reviewed by Dr. Grollman. Particular attention was focused on recently identified DNA intermediates that could participate in the cellular toxicity. The basic histological and biochemical aspects of interstitial fibrosis of the lung were summarized by Drs. Tryka and Kelley. The complete morphologic manifestation of both the acute and chronic phases of the disease was presented as was a comparison between high oxygen and bleomycin-induced disease states. Dr. Kelley addressed the immunologic mechanisms responsible for the generation of drug-induced fibrosis as well as the effects of bleomycin on specific pulmonary cell types in the lung, such as macrophages.

The manifestations of cellular toxicity in the lungs and the biochemical basis for the injury were the focus of Drs. Catravas and Lazo. The pulmonary capillary endothelium is an early target of damage, and new means to reveal the injury in vivo and with cultured cells were summarized. The role of metabolic inactivation of the bleomycins by the enzyme bleomycin hydrolase also was reviewed. In addition, recent results that provide information on the biochemical and molecular nature of this enzyme were presented.

One biochemical approach to blocking bleomycin-induced fibrosis was reviewed by Dr. Cutroneo: glucocorticoids, which affect the deposition of extracellular matrix components, such as collagen. These studies form a conceptual framework for future experiments designed to develop novel means to prevent drug-induced fibrosis. The recent improvements in our understanding of the basic pathogenesis of pulmonary fibrosis and the cellular and biochemical changes that ensue should provide the foundation for new approaches to detect the onset of lung injury and to develop pharmacologic agents to prevent and possibly reverse this disease.

Base Propenals and the Toxicity of Bleomycin
A.P. Grollman

INTRODUCTION

It is generally believed that bleomycin-induced degradation of DNA leads to inhibition of DNA synthesis and that these effects are jointly responsible for the cytotoxic properties of this antibiotic (1,2). However, a direct relationship between DNA damage, inhibition of DNA synthesis and cytotoxicity has not been established and several reports exist in the literature which cast doubt on this fundamental hypothesis. For example, bleomycin-induced DNA damage apparently can be repaired (3); nevertheless, cells in culture treated with bleomycin frequently do not survive, suggesting involvement of lethal factors other than strand scission. Moore (4) reported that yeast are more susceptible to killing when incubated with cells previously treated with bleomycin and proposed the intermediacy of a diffusible toxic product. Cohen and I (5) found that bacterial killing by bleomycin occurs at concentrations of drug that do not affect DNA synthesis.

Further questions are raised by the effects of bleomycin when introduced at various times during the cell cycle. Most drugs which block DNA synthesis act almost exclusively during S phase (6). Bleomycin, however, inhibits cell growth during G2 phase near the S/G2 boundary and cells treated in S or G1 phase recover following antibiotic-induced damage (7,8). Selective impairment of enzymes or other proteins involved in mitotic functions might account for these observations.

In this paper, I will summarize evidence supporting the view (9,10) that some, or possibly all, of the cellular toxicity of bleomycin can be attributed to intermediates formed during the degradation of DNA by bleomycin. Implications of this hypothesis for the development of bleomycin analogs will be discussed.

BLEOMYCIN AND DNA DAMAGE

The mechanism by which bleomycin binds to and cleaves DNA has been elucidated, primarily through the studies of Grollman, Haidle, Hecht, Horwitz, Kozarich, Peisach, Povirk, Sugiura, Takeshita, Takita, Umezawa and their associates (1,2). A molecular model for the bleomycin-Fe(II)-O_2-DNA complex has been proposed (11), the principal features of which involve coordination of molecular oxygen to the metal and preferential intercalation of bithiazole rings at GpT and GpC sequences (Fig. 1). Binding of bleomycin is stabilized through electrostatic interactions between the positively-charged terminal side chain of the drug and the negatively-charged phosphate group on the opposite strand of DNA. The oxygen molecule in this complex is positioned strategically so that, upon reduction to a radical species, the 4' hydrogen atom of deoxyribose is abstracted selectively.

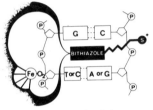

Fig. 1 Schematic representation of the bleomycin Fe(II)-O_2-DNA complex.

Treatment with bleomycin alters the structure of DNA in several ways. Apurinic and apyridiminic sites arise in the absence of strand breaks (12). Strand-scission is associated with the production of oligodeoxynucleotides containing O-phosphoglycolate residues at the 3' terminus (13).

Several low molecular weight products are produced during the degradation of DNA by bleomycin. In the presence of molecular oxygen, base propenals and free heterocyclic bases are released (13). In the absence of oxygen, only free bases are found (14). Base propenals and free bases appear to originate from attack at the C-4' position of deoxyribose. A mechanism for this reaction has been proposed (9).

Double-strand breaks, occuring at AP sites and/or the site of deoxyribose cleavage, represent potentially lethal cellular events. As noted in the Introduction to this paper and in critical reviews of the subject (1,2), the direct relationship between DNA damage and cytotoxicity has been questioned. Drugs that promote the formation of oxygen radicals may lead to tissue damage (15) and, in the absence of DNA, the bleomycin-Fe(II)-O_2 complex can generate reactive oxygen species (16). However, in a cellular environment, bleomycin exists as a stable copper complex which is incapable of generating free radicals under physiological conditions (2). When bound to DNA, the only demonstrated radical-forming reaction of bleomycin-Fe(II)O_2 involves the direct abstraction of a proton from the deoxyribose moiety of DNA (13). In this case, damage is initially limited to the DNA molecule.

Bleomycin cleaves DNA in a site-specific manner (17-19), provided that the target sequences are not protected by complexation to proteins. Oligodeoxynucleotide fragments, produced by the action of the antibiotic, are resistant to degradation by intracellular phosphatases and are inactive as templates for DNA polymerase I (20). Thus, in the absence of DNA repair, genes critical to cell survival may be directly inactivated by bleomycin. DNA synthesis is interrupted when replicative DNA polymerases encounter strand breaks, AP sites or 3' glycolate termini created by the drug.

CHEMISTRY OF BASE PROPENALS

Base propenals are electrophiles which readily undergo addition-elimination reactions with primary amino or thiol groups (9,21). These substances are also capable of forming Schiff bases and cyclic amino-acetals. The heterocylic base moiety of the base propenals is an excellent leaving group, a property that seems not to have been widely recognized. At physiological pH, rates of these reactions vary considerably, proceeding rapidly with β-mercaptoethanol and glutathione and more slowly with primary amines (21).

Base propenals undergo 1,4-addition reactions with nucleophiles and are likely to exert their biological activity by reacting with sulfhydryl or amino functions of critical macromolecules. Behaving essentially as reversible alkylating agents, these compounds may enter into 1,2-addition reactions to form diadducts; this mechanism could lead to crosslinking reactions and condensation with amino groups.

In effect, base propenals represent masked forms of malonaldehyde. As such, they are more reactive than free malonaldehyde which exists as a highly-stabilized anion in aqueous solution. Thus, base propenals readily form adducts under physiological conditions with simple nucleophiles such as glutathione (9), and β-mercaptoethanol (13).

BASE PROPENALS AND THE CYTOXICITY OF BLEOMYCIN

Bleomycin generates several potentially toxic products from DNA, including damaged DNA and base propenals (9). The latter, formed in conjunction with DNA strand breaks, inhibit macromolecular synthesis in HeLa cells and are highly toxic to tumor cells in culture (9). We have suggested (9,10) that these activities may be responsible for some or all of the toxic and/or chemotherapeutic effects of the antibiotic. Our proposal is based, in part, on the well-established cytotoxic properties of other α,β unsaturated aldehydes. Substances bearing this functional group have been implicated as environmental toxins and mutagens (22,23) and shown to be powerful inhibitors of cellular enzymes (22).

Base propenals, generated in the nucleus by the action of bleomycin, could react under physiological conditions to form adducts with proteins and/or DNA. Undoubtedly, such complexes would be deleterious to cellular functions. Base propenals are precursors of malonaldehyde, a naturally-occurring product of lipid peroxidation, which also reacts with DNA (24).

There is general agreement that therapeutic concentrations of bleomycin preferentially inhibit DNA synthesis in cultured cells (1,2). Inhibition of macromolecular synthesis in HeLa cells by bleomycin (25) is qualitatively and quantitatively similar to effects observed in cells treated with base propenals (9). Based on the proposed mechanism of action (9,10), stoichiometric amounts of base propenals should be formed for each mole of bleomycin involved in strand scission. These substances, presumably liberated during strand scission of DNA, could inactivate sulfhydryl-containing enzymes in the cell nucleus, including those involved with DNA synthesis.

Pulmonary fibrosis is an important toxic effect of bleomycin in man. An enzyme activity, bleomycin hydrolase, has been described (26) which inactivates bleomycin in various organs and is absent from lung and skin, insuring that higher concentrations of the antibiotic and, therefore, base propenals, would accumulate in these tissues (27). We postulate that liberation of base propenals and their subsequent reaction with proteins or enzymes contributes to this pathological process.

Most of the cytotoxic effects of bleomycin can be satisfactorily explained on the basis of intranuclear generation of cytotoxic base propenals. Breaks, gaps, deletions and other chromosomal abberations have also been reported to occur in bleomycin-treated cells (3) and the DNA damage produced may contribute to the overall cytotoxicity of the drug.

INHIBITION OF DNA SYNTHESIS

Base propenals inhibit synthesis of DNA in cultured cells (21). We have tested the effects of these compounds on each of the several steps involved in this critical process. Thymidine kinase and DNA polymerase were selectively inhibited by thymidine-3-N-propenal, a synthetic base propenal containing the deoxyribose ring (9). In contrast, these two enzyme activities were only weakly inhibited by the base propenals generated by the action of bleomycin on DNA. Recently, we tested the effect of thymine-N-propenal on the activity of thymidylate synthetase in permeabilized L1210 and L-cells. Using an assay based on tritium release from the 5-position of dUMP, thymidylate synthetase was inhibited by 50% at concentrations of <10 µM (Kalman, Marinelli, Xu, Johnson and Grollman, unpublished studies). Reduction of the unsaturated aldehyde group abolished this inhibitory activity.

BASE SPECIFICITY AND DRUG DESIGN

The bleomycins comprise a group of metallo-glycopeptides differing in their terminal amine side chain (28). Phleomycins are structurally related to bleomycins, differing in that one of the thiazole rings is partially saturated. Tallysomycins resemble bleomycins but contain an additional amino-sugar moiety and a methyl group linked to the backbone of the molecule.

Despite significant structural differences, all bleomycins, phleomycins and talisomycins thus far tested display similar specificity towards DNA; namely, they cleave preferentially GC (5'—>3') and GT (5'—>3') sequences in DNA, releasing the pyrimidine base (17-19). Phleomycin analogs show less preference for binding to purines than do bleomycins and cleave purine-purine sequences with low frequency. These observations may reflect steric problems encountered by the partly nonplanar phleomycin ring in forming an intercalation complex. Marked differences in base specificity between the bleomycin antibiotics are not observed, suggesting that the side chain containing the terminal amine, which represents the only structural difference between these analogs, does not contribute significantly to the base-specificity of the cleavage reaction.

Assuming that double-strand breaks are the result of closely-spaced single-strand scissions on opposite strands, base-specificity of bleomycin for double-strand DNA is represented by several tetra-, penta- and hexa-nucleotide consensus sequences (19). This conclusion is consistent with the observations of Lloyd et al. (29) who reported that low concentrations of bleomycin produce double-strand breaks in plasmid DNA at a limited number of discrete sites. This confers on bleomycin a degree of base specificity associated with certain restriction enzymes.

Considerable efforts have been made to modify the side chains of bleomycin, phleomycin and tallysomycin so as to enhance their therapeutic activity and to minimize the pulmonary and renal toxicities caused by these drugs (28,30). Base-specific cleavage of DNA is not markedly altered by these structural changes; thus, modification of the side chains can be expected to primarily alter transport and organ distribution.

Synthetic analogs of bleomycin have been designed, based on the premise that DNA cleavage underlies the therapeutic actions of the drug (31,32). Unfortunately, this strategy tends to overlook the possibility that the cellular mechanism responsible for the therapeutic properties of bleomycin may be identical with that which leads to its toxic actions. If this premise proves correct, development of more effective analogs with similar sequence specificity for DNA should focus on structural changes which alter pharmacokinetic properties and organ distribution of the drug. Structure-activity relationships governing cellular uptake and transport of bleomycin are predictably different from those which affect cleavage of DNA; the recent development of libleomycin (cf 30) may prove to be a case in point.

This basic tenet of drug development is exemplified by earlier investigations of the cardiac glycosides, a class of drugs which exert inotropic (therapeutic) and arrythmogenic (toxic) effects by inhibiting the activity of the Na/K ATP'ase located in the cardiac membrane. Many new cardiac glycosides, exhibiting a wide range of therapeutic activities, have been discovered over the years. Although these compounds vary widely in their absorption, excretion and organ distribution, no significant improvement in therapeutic ratio has yet emerged.

SUMMARY AND CONCLUSIONS

Cytotoxicity reflects the chemotherapeutic potential of bleomycin and underlies its principal side effect, pulmonary fibrosis. Several lines of evidence suggest that DNA strand scission alone may not account fully for the cytotoxic effects of this drug. An important clue is provided by the identification of nucleoside base-N-propenals produced by the action of bleomycin on DNA. Base propenals inhibit DNA synthesis and are highly cytotoxic when added to tumor cells in culture. We propose that these unsaturated aldehydes, generated in the cell nucleus, inhibit critical cellular enzymes, thereby accounting for the cytostatic and cytotoxic properties of bleomycin. This hypothesis has implications for the design of bleomycin analogs. If the basic mechanism responsible for the therapeutic and toxic properties is identical, development of bleomycin analogs with similar sequence specificity for DNA, should effectively concentrate on structural modifications which might alter pharmacokinetic properties and organ distribution of the drug.

ACKNOWLEDGEMENTS

The many contributions of Masaru Takeshita and Francis Johnson to the experiments and ideas discussed in this paper, are gratefully acknowledged.

REFERENCES

1. Haidle, C.W., and Lloyd, R.S. (1979) In: Antibiotics: Mechanism of Action of Antieukaryotic and Antiviral Compounds. Ed. Hahn, F.E., (Springer-Verlag, New York), pp. 123-154.
2. Povirk, L.F. (1983) In: Molecular Aspects of Anti-Cancer Drug Action. Eds. Neidle, S. and Waring, M.J., (McMillan Press, New York), pp. 157-181.
3. Vig, B.K., and Lewis, R. (1978) Mutation Res. 55, 121-145.
4. Moore, C.W. (1982) Antimicrob. Agents and Chemotherapy 21: 595-600.
5. Cohen, S. and I, J. (1976) Cancer Res. 36: 2768-2774.
6. Hoffman, J. and Post, J. (1973) In: Drugs and the Cell Cycle. Eds. Zimmerman, T.M., Padilla, G.D. and Cameron, I.L. (Academic Press, New York), pp. 219-247.
7. Barranco, S.C. (1978) In: Bleomycin: Current Status and New Developments. Eds. Carter, S.K., Crooke, S.T. and Umezawa, H. (Academic Press, New York), pp. 81-90.

8. Twentyman, P.R. (1984) Pharmacol. Ther. $\underline{23}$: 417-441.
9. Grollman, A.P, Takeshita, M., Pillai, K.M.R. and Johnson, F. (1985) Cancer Res. $\underline{45}$, 1127-1131.
10. Johnson, F. and Grollman, A.P. (1985) In: Experimental and Clinical Progress in Cancer Chemotherapy. Ed: Muggia, F.M. (Martinus Nijhoff Publishers, Boston), pp. 1-12.
11. Takeshita, M. and Grollman, A.P. (1980) In: Advances in Enzyme Regulation $\underline{18}$, Ed: Weber, G., (Pergamon Press), pp. 673-683.
12. Ross, S.L. and Moses, R.E. (1978) Biochemistry $\underline{17}$: 581-586.
13. Giloni, L., Takeshita, M., Johnson, F., Iden, C. and Grollman, A.P. (1981) J. Biol. Chem. $\underline{256}$: 8606-8615.
14. Burger, R.M., Peisach, J. and Horwitz, S.B. (1982) J. Biol. Chem. $\underline{257}$: 3372-3375.
15. Trush, M.A., Mimnaugh, E.G. and Gram, T.E. (1982) Biochem. Pharm. $\underline{31}$: 3335-3346.
16. Caspary, W.J., Niziak, C., Lanzo, D.A., Friedman, R. and Bachur, N.R. (1979) Molec. Pharm. $\underline{16}$: 256-260.
17. Takeshita, M., Grollman, A.P., Ohtsubo, E. and Ohtsubo, H. (1978) Proc. Natl. Acad. Sci. $\underline{75}$: 5983-5987.
18. D'Andrea, D.D. and Hazeltine, W.A. (1978) Proc. Natl. Acad. Sci. USA $\underline{75}$: 3608-3612.
19. Takeshita, M., Kappen, L.S., Grollman, A.P., Eisenberg, M. and Goldberg, I.H. (1981) Biochemistry $\underline{20}$: 7599-7606.
20. Niwa, O. and Moses, R.E. (1981) Biochemistry $\underline{20}$: 238-243.
21. Johnson, F., Pillai, K.M.R., Grollman, A.P., Tseng, L., Takeshita, M. (1984) J. Med. Chem. $\underline{27}$: 954-958.
22. Schauenstein, E., Esterbauer, H. and Zollner, H. (1977) In: Aldehydes in Biological Systems: Their Natural Occurrence and Biological Activities, (Pion Press, London), pp. 25-102
23. Eder, E., Henschler, D. and Neudecker, T. (1982) Xenobiotica $\underline{12}$: 831-848.
24. Brooks, B.R and Klamerth, O.L. (1968) European J. Biochem. $\underline{5}$: 178-182.
25. Takeshita, M., Horwitz, S.B. and Grollman, A.P. (1974) Virology $\underline{60}$: 455-465.
26. Umezawa, H., Takeuchi, T., Hori, S., Sawa, T., Ishizuka, M., Ichikawa, T. and Kanai, T. (1972) J. Antibiot $\underline{25}$: 409-420.
27. Lazo, J. and Humphreys, C.J. (1983) Proc. Natl. Acad. Sci. $\underline{80}$: 3064-3068.
28. Umezawa, H. (1977) Lloydia $\underline{40}$: 67-81.

29. Lloyd, R.S., Haidle, C.W. and Robberson, D.L. (1978) Biochemistry 17: 1890-1896.
30. Umezawa, H. et. al. (1985) In: Bleomycin Chemotherapy. Eds Sikic, B.I., Rozencweig, M. and Carter, S.K. (Academic Press, New York), pp. 289-301.
31. Sugiura, Y. et. al. (1983) J. Biol. Chem. 258: 1328-1336.
32. Dervan, P.B. (1986) Science 232: 464-471.

Bleomycin Induced Lung Injury
A.F. Tryka

INTRODUCTION

Bleomycin is a highly effective cytotoxic antibiotic, whose clinical use is limited by pulmonary toxicity. The reported risk of developing pulmonary toxicity varies widely, from 2 to 40% (1). Risk factors in developing toxicity include age, cumulative dose, use with other cytotoxic drugs, radiation therapy and oxygen (1). The most frequent manifestation of bleomycin induced pulmonary injury is the development of a diffuse alveolar damage frequently followed by interstitial fibrosis (2), although hypersensitivity reactions have been reported (3). This chapter will focus on the morphologic aspects of bleomycin induced interstitial pulmonary disease. The mechanisms implicated in bleomycin induced pneumonitis will be summarized. The histologic lesions seen in both the acute and chronic phases of the disease will be discussed. Results of study of experimental bleomycin induced pulmonary disease will be presented, including cell kinetics, potentiation of the disease by oxygen, and implications of these studies on the understanding of the underlying mechanisms which dictate development of the fibrosis.

MECHANISMS OF LUNG INJURY

The mechanisms whereby pneumotoxic agents may

injure the lung may be broadly grouped into three categories. These are 1) direct toxic effect on lung cells, 2) effects of circulating leukocytes, and 3) production and release of endogenous chemical mediators. There is evidence to suggest that each of these three mechanisms may play a role in the development of bleomycin induced lung injury.

Pneumotoxic agents may directly injure the alveolar cells by damaging the cell membrane, by poisoning the cellular metabolic machinery, or by production of highly reactive free radicals. If this injury targets the epithelial cells lining the alveolus, the alveolar surface is denuded of cells and the type II pneumocytes may not be able to produce surfactant. This would result in alveolar collapse, and failure of gas exchange in the affected region. If endothelial cells are damaged, the capillaries leak their contents into the alveolar spaces, a situation which also results in a failure of gas exchange. The classic example of an agent which is directly toxic to cells is oxygen. Oxygen exerts its effects by the generation of highly reactive free radicals (4).

Bleomycin may also exert its toxic effect by generating reactive oxygen metabolites. Bleomycin has been reported to generate superoxide anions when incubated in vitro with iron in the presence of oxygen (5). The oxidation of the Fe(II)-bleomycin-DNA complex is postulated to be the etiology of the DNA damage caused by bleomycin (5).

Circulating leukocytes play an important role in mediating lung injury. This effect may be a result of 1) passive accumulation of leukocytes in the pulmonary vasculature, or 2) by actual recruitment to the lung. In the former, leukocytes may be injured directly by the chemical agent. Since all the blood passes through the lung in transit to the systemic circulation, cells within the blood including leukocytes must pass through the pulmonary capillary bed. If the cell surface of leukocytes becomes altered from injury, these cells will tend to aggregate when brought into the close proximity of one another within these small caliber vessels, and be trapped in the lung. In the second mechanism, leukocytes may accumulate in the lung by responding to injury. This form of aggregation within the pulmonary vasculature is an integral part of the body's defense mechanism, as well as a part of the healing response. In performing this role in injury and repair, leukocytes respond to cell injury or to released chemotactic factors. In either of these two modes of accumulation, leukocytes may cause injury by their mere presence in the lung. Neutrophils contain cytoplasmic enzymes such as collagenase, elastase, and lysozyme. Leakage of these potent cytoplasmic enzymes occurs passively during the process of endocytosis, or by release of cytoplasmic contents when the cell is injured. Neutrophils also generate superoxides. These agents may in themselves result in cellular injury or may compound preexisting cell injury. Monocytes and lymphocytes may behave similarly, although their cytoplasmic enzymes are considered less potent.

There is considerable evidence that bleomycin injured cells are chemotactic for neutrophils. Release of chemotactic substances for neutrophils from the supernatant of cells obtained by bronchoalveolar lavage in experimental animals has been demonstrated (6-8).

A third mechanism of lung injury is production of endogenously produced chemicals, which in themselves may mediate lung injury. Examples include complement, arachidonic acid, prostaglandins and leukotrienes. The later three have been implicated in bleomycin lung injury (7). These chemicals, which have a normal physiologic role, may also play a role in lung injury when their action is inappropriately triggered. Many of these mediators act as a chemoattractant or otherwise trap circulating leukocytes in the lung.

HISTOPATHOLOGY OF BLEOMYCIN INDUCED LUNG DISEASE

Study of experimental bleomycin lung injury has provided an opportunity to enhance the understanding of interstitial lung disease. The early pulmonary effects of bleomycin treatment results in the histopathologic lesion termed diffuse alveolar damage (DAD). DAD is the lung's stereotypic response to alveolar injury and is the morphologic manifestation of acute respiratory distress syndrome (ARDS) (9). The appearance of DAD reflects both injury and the dynamic process of repair. Because injury always initiates a repair response, the morphology of a particular lesion depends, in part, by the duration of time passed after the inciting event. Diffuse alveolar damage can be divided into two phases, the 1) exudative, and 2) the proliferative phase (9).

The exudative phase is observed the first week after treatment with bleomycin. It is characterized by interstitial edema, sloughing of alveolar lining cells and on occasion, hyaline membranes. The exudative phase is the result of injury to either the endothelial cell or the type II pneumocyte. With damage to these cells, there is a loss of integrity of the vascular compartment, with resultant leakage of serum constituents into the interstitial and alveolar space.

The proliferative phase, which commences the second week after treatment, reflects the repair process of the lung. There is a increase in the number of type II pneumocytes, which reflects the role of this cell as progenitor of alveolar epithelial regeneration. The alveolar wall appears thick (Figure 1), due to both an infiltrate of inflammatory cells, and the continued presence of interstitial edema. There may also be an influx of fibroblasts into the alveolar airspace, in an aberrant attempt to organize intraalveolar material. Depending on the severity of the initial injury and the success of the repair process seen in the proliferative phase, the lung may heal with little residual scarring, or as in the case with bleomycin, more frequently interstitial pulmonary fibrosis develops.

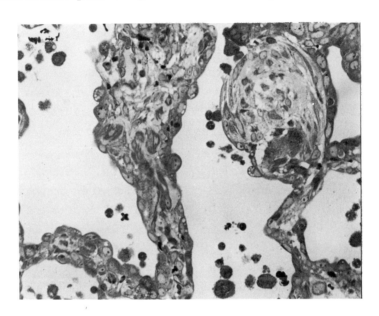

Figure 1.   Proliferative phase of diffuse alveolar damage.

EXPERIMENTAL BLEOMYCIN INDUCED LUNG INJURY

In experimental studies on the pathogenesis of bleomycin induced lung disease, the intratracheal method of instilling the drug is frequently used. Intratracheal administration is a convenient and reproducible method to expose the lung to a high concentration of bleomycin. Use of the intravascular or intraperitoneal route requires considerably higher doses of drug and may result in significant morbidity in other organ systems to achieve a marked degree of fibrosis. Since the intratracheal route may in theory result in initial injury to the epithelium, while a systemic dose may initially damage the endothelium, there is a theoretical concern that these routes of exposure may fail to be equivalent in terms of the injury response.

We performed a study to answer the question, is there a difference in the pulmonary response between intratracheal (IT) or intravenous (IV) administration of bleomycin (10). Mice were treated with either 4U/kg IT or 100U/Kg IV. These doses should result in approximately equivalent bleomycin levels in the lung, based on radiolabeled bleomycin studies (11). Cell kinetics, histopathology, lung lavage enzyme levels, and total lung hydroxyproline content were analyzed.

Cell kinetic studies were accomplished by utilizing autoradiographic histologic slides. This method permits morphologic evaluation, as well as a quantitative measure of which cells are preparing to undergo cell division. The results are expressed as the labeling index, the number of cells labeled/total number of cells counted.

Mice treated with IV bleomycin demonstrated a depression of the labeling index the first several days after treatment. Then a sharp rise in the labeling index was observed 13 days after treatment, which peaked on day 17, and returned to control values by day 21 (10).

Intratracheal administration of bleomycin resulted in an initial sharp peak in the overall labeling index, 5 days after treatment. An early rise in the IT saline treated controls was also observed, and probably reflects a non-specific response to the presence of migrating inflammatory cells reacting to the instillation (12). A second rise in the labeling index, in the bleomycin treated animals, occurred on day 9. The labeling index then remained elevated until 17 days after treatment (10). This elevation in the labeling index observed in both groups in the second week after treatment, correlates with the proliferative phase of diffuse alveolar damage. The labeled cells were further differentiated into the four alveolar cell types counted, endothelial, interstitial, epithelial pneumocyte and macrophages. There were no differences in the patterns of the elevations of the specific cell type between the IV and IT treatments (10).

Activities of lactate dehydrogenase (LDH), alkaline phosphatase, acid phosphatase and angiotensin converting enzyme from bronchoalveolar lavage fluid were examined (10). There was an elevation of LDH in both the IV and IT treated mice during most of the study period. Alkaline phosphatase, an enzyme detected in the type II pneumocyte, was elevated in both groups at days 11-17. Acid phosphatase, derived from phagocytic cells, was markedly elevated in both groups at days 11-17. Angiotensin converting enzyme activity was elevated during most of the study period. This analysis showed similar patterns of enzyme release by the two routes of administration. Total lung hydroxyproline content, measured three weeks after treatment, was elevated in both treatment groups, although the IT treated animals demonstrated higher total levels (10).

Comparison of the two routes of bleomycin administration, intravenous verses intratracheal, reveals basic similarities in the acute reaction of the lung. Histologically, the lesions observed in both treatment groups was a interstitial pneumonitis. In both routes of administration, the onset of resolution of the injury, as determined by histologic interpretation, appeared at approximately the same time (day 15). Analysis of the bronchoalveolar lavage showed similar patterns of enzyme elevation in the two routes of administration. Differences between the two routes of administration included an earlier and more elevated alveolar cell proliferation in the intratracheally instilled animals. Also, total hydroxyproline content was higher in these animals. However, these differences may be attributed to differences in severity of the initial damage and a nonspecific response to the intratracheal route of administration.

POTENTIATION OF BLEOMYCIN INDUCED LUNG INJURY BY OXYGEN

Oxygen alone can result in diffuse alveolar damage, and is reported to be a risk factor in the development of bleomycin induced lung injury. The possibility of interaction between the two pneumotoxic agents, bleomycin and hyperoxia, was first suggested in a clinical report. Goldiner and coworkers (13) reported 5 young men treated with bleomycin for testicular carcinoma, who later underwent a staging laparotomy. All 5 unexpectedly developed respiratory failure and died postoperatively. The investigators implicated either an elevated inspired oxygen concentration (>0.39) or excess intravenous fluids. More cautious fluid replacement and a mean FIO_2 of 0.24 in the next 12 patients resulted in uneventful postoperative courses.

Potentiation of bleomycin induced lung injury by hyperoxia was investigated in hamsters (14). Hamsters were initially treated with a single intratracheal instillation of 5U/Kg of bleomycin. This treatment resulted in a 15%- 30 day cumulative mortality. If hamsters were exposed to 70% oxygen for 72 hours immediately after the 5U/Kg dose of bleomycin, deaths occurred much earlier, at 4 days, and the cumulative mortality was 90%. There was no mortality in the hyperoxia alone treated animals. Multiple lower doses were examined and the data from this study are illustrated in the dose response curve in Figure 2. The LD50 for a single intratracheal instillation of bleomycin was 7.3U/Kg, with a 95% confidence interval of

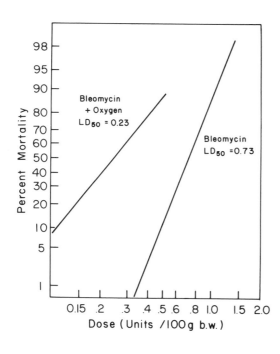

6.7 and 8.1. However, the LD50 in hamsters treated with bleomycin and hyperoxia was a much lower 2.3U/Kg, with the 95% confidence interval of 1.8 and 2.8. Also, there was a significant difference in the slopes of the two curves, suggesting a different mechanism of action of the two agents.

Figure 2. Dose response plot (Reprinted with permission from ref. 14).

The concomitant treatment with bleomycin and hyperoxia also resulted in greater amounts of lung demonstrating disease. The resulting interstitial pneumonitis and fibrosis present one month after bleomycin treatment was quantitatively evaluated utilizing morphometric methods. The amount of lung which was diseased increased dramatically in the bleomycin and hyperoxia treated hamsters. After treatment with 2U/Kg of bleomycin alone, 2.8±1.6% of the lung was diseased, but with 2U/Kg bleomycin followed by exposure to 70% oxygen for 72h, 42.7% of the lung was abnormal. This marked increase in lung disease indicates a synergistic effect, rather than simply an additive effect. This synergistic effect is most evident at low doses of bleomycin. Virtually no lesions were seen in the animals treated with 1.6U/Kg bleomycin alone or with saline and hyperoxia. However, when these 2 treatments were combined, a significant (10.6%) amount of disease was observed. This demonstrates the potential for even moderate amounts of hyperoxia to enhance the lung damaging effects of bleomycin at doses where changes would not be expected.

What is the minimum duration of exposure to hyperoxia which will result in this synergistic effect? To answer this question, hamsters were treated with 5U/Kg of bleomycin. Then groups of animals were exposed to either 12, 24, 48, 72 or 96 hours of 80% oxygen. As little as 12 hours of hyperoxia exposure resulted in an increased mortality in the bleomycin treated animals (15). However, exposure to 6 hours of hyperoxia fails to increase mortality (Tryka, unpublished observations).

Although apparent irreversible injury occurred within 12 hours, the onset of mortality was delayed until 72 hours after treatment (15). Additionally, the onset of mortality was similar irrespective of whether the animal was exposed to hyperoxia only 12 hours or to various intervals up to continuous. The development of alveolar edema, as measured by radiolabeled tracers, was examined in hamsters treated with 5U/Kg bleomycin followed by 24-h exposure to 80% oxygen. Alveolar edema was only initially detectable 72 hours post initial bleomycin treatment (15). However, interstitial edema could be detected on histologic examination of the tissue much earlier, at 24 hours after bleomycin treatment.

The acute phase of bleomycin and hyperoxia injury was also examined utilizing autoradiography. Hamsters treated with 5U/Kg of bleomycin followed by 24 hour exposure to 80% oxygen were sacrificed 24, 48, 72 or 96 hours after treatment. Significant increase in total cell labeling was seen only at 96h post treatment in the bleomycin and air, and in the bleomycin and hyperoxia treated animals. A slight decrease in total cell labeling at 72 hours in the oxygen treated hamsters, which returned to control values at 96 hours was also observed (15). When the labeled cells were differentiated into individual cell types, the labeling of the endothelial, interstitial cells and macrophages were found to be similar between the bleomycin alone, and bleomycin and hyperoxia treated animals. However, the addition of hyperoxia exposure to the bleomycin treatment resulted in a depression of the increased type II pneumocyte labeling seen the in bleomycin alone treated animals (Figure 3).

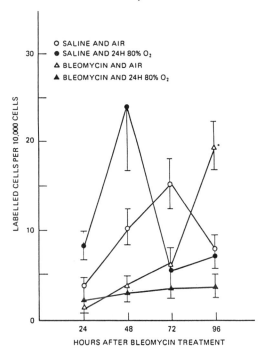

Figure 3. Type II pneumocyte labeling in hamsters treated with 5.0U/Kg bleomycin followed by 24h exposure to 80% oxygen (Redrawn with permission from ref. 15).

DELAYED OXYGEN EXPOSURE IN BLEOMYCIN INJURED LUNGS

While concomitant treatment with bleomycin and hyperoxia results in a synergistic effect on the resultant lung injury, is there a similar effect when hyperoxia exposure is delayed until the lung has healed from the bleomycin injury? To examine this question, hamsters were treated with 5U/Kg of bleomycin. One or two months after the bleomycin treatment, the hamsters were exposed to either 70 or 100% oxygen for 72 hours, then observed for mortality over the following month. There was no increase in mortality between the bleomycin and the bleomycin and hyperoxia treated groups (16). Also, morphometric evaluation of the lungs failed to reveal a significant difference in the amount of lung disease observed (16). In conclusion, although concomitant treatment with bleomycin and hyperoxia results in a synergistic effect on the development of pulmonary toxicity, if the hyperoxia exposure is delayed until the bleomycin induced lesions have healed (1 month in hamsters), there is no increased susceptibility to oxygen toxicity.

PROGRESSIVE PULMONARY FIBROSIS

Thus far this chapter has focused on the acute phase of bleomycin induced lung injury. In animals treated with bleomycin alone, the diffuse alveolar damage lesions are healed by one month after treatment, leaving a focal residual pulmonary fibrosis. This form of pulmonary fibrosis is relevant to the form of lung disease termed acute respiratory distress syndrome (ARDS). ARDS is a syndrome which has an acute onset, and in which the clinical course events is measured in weeks.

Another form of pulmonary fibrosis occurs where the initiating event is silent. The patient presents with cough and dyspnea, and the histologic finding in the lung is interstitial pneumonitis with a variable amount of histologically identified interstitial fibrosis. The time course of this disease is long, occurring over a period of months to years (17). I propose that if one looks at animals treated with a low dose of bleomycin and hyperoxia, one will find a second phase of progressive fibrosis in these animals (18,19).

Sprague dawley rats were treated with 1.6U/Kg

bleomycin, then exposed to 70% oxygen for 72 hours. Animals were killed at 15, 30, 60 and 90 days after treatment. Their lungs were evaluated for hydroxyproline content, cell kinetics and morphometrically for cellularity. The results from the hydroxyproline analysis are presented in Table 1.

Table 1

days after treatment	15	30	60	90
bleo-O_2	4945± 147[a]	5248± 340[a]	5133± 246[a]	6238± 257[b]
bleo-air	4731± 151[a]	4603± 117	4356± 109	4719± 168
saline-O_2	4569± 92	4568± 210	4387± 89	4840± 189
saline-a	4366± 169	4360± 196	4509± 109	4500± 131

[a] Significantly increased over saline-air controls.
[b] Significantly increased over both controls and increased levels seen in bleo-O_2 60 day animals.

There was a significant increase in total lung hydroxyproline content in the bleomycin and hyperoxia treated rats 15 days after treatment, which remained elevated through 60 days. At 90 days, there was a second significant increase, over the increased values observed at 60 days. A transient increase in hydroxyproline levels was observed only at 15 days in the bleomycin and air treated rats. Cell kinetics revealed a significant increase in labeling in the bleomycin and hyperoxia treated rats at 15 days. By 30 days, the cell labeling returned to control values, and remained there through the 90 day study. There was a consistent increase in cellularity, as assessed by morphometric methods, in the bleomycin and hyperoxia animals throughout the study (18).

This study reaffirmed previous findings described in hamsters (19), that treatment with a combination of bleomycin and hyperoxia results in a slowly progressive pulmonary fibrosis. Further, it was observed that between 60 and the 90 day time-point, when hydroxyproline levels were continuing to increase, there was no increase in cell proliferation or total number of lung cells. Thus, we concluded that during this slowly progressive phase, there was an increase in the amount of collagen being produced by the interstitial cells, not an increase in the total number of cells producing a unit amount of collagen.

CONCLUSIONS

In the first section of this chapter, mechanisms of lung injury were divided into three categories. Which of these mechanisms, 1) direct toxic effect, 2) circulating leukocytes, or 3) endogenous mediators, best explains the injury seen in bleomycin induced pulmonary disease? The most frequently cited putative mechanism is the production of free radicals, which would point to the direct toxic effect mechanism. However, oxygen, which unquestionably exerts its effect by free radical injury to cells, fails to result in a significant degree of residual lung disease, unless the exposure is continuous. Bleomycin apparently continues to exert its effect long after the drug is metabolized and cleared.

Experimental studies, some presented in this chapter, of the potentiation of bleomycin induced lung injury indicate that there may be different mechanisms responsible for the two agents, bleomycin and oxygen. The difference in the slope of the dose response curves (Figure 2), suggests different mechanisms of action. Bleomycin and hyperoxia treatment results in a slowly progressive pulmonary fibrosis, which develops over several months (18,19), which differs from the healed lesion seen in the bleomycin alone treated animals (19). Cell labeling in acute injury demonstrates a suppression of type II pneumocyte labeling when oxygen was added to bleomycin treatment (15). The failure of this cell to cover the denuded alveolar epithelial surface and participate in contact with fibroblasts, basement membrane, and collagen has been postulated to be an important factor in development of pulmonary fibrosis (20). Close examination of lesions seen in animals three days after treatment with bleomycin and hyperoxia, bleomycin alone, or hyperoxia alone, indicates that a qualitative difference can be observed, in addition to the alteration in cell labeling detected by autoradiography. The lesions of oxygen exposed animals are mostly edematous in nature with little inflammation observable (19). With bleomycin and hyperoxia, or bleomycin alone, in addition to interstitial edema, there is a significant infiltrate of inflammatory cells observed, including neutrophils and mononuclear cells (19). These observations would indicate that the bleomycin lesion is mediated through the effects of circulating leukocytes that have accumulated in the lungs. The initiating event for this aggregation may be direct cell injury, or even mild cell damage insufficient to cause cell death. Either of these events may result in the release of endogenous mediators which may in fact be responsible for the recruitment of the inflammatory cells.

In conclusion, I propose that careful histologic observation coupled with correlation with the clinical manifestations of lung disease, will lead to an improved understanding of pulmonary interstitial disease. The study of the synergistic effect of bleomycin and hyperoxia has enhanced this understanding of the mechanisms of lung disease. Morphologic observation will also play an integral role in determining the effectiveness of pharmacologic alterations of bleomycin induced lung disease.

REFERENCES

1. Cooper JAD, White DA, Matthay RA. (1986) Am Rev Respir Dis 133:321-40.
2. Luna MA, et al. (1972) Am J Clin Path 58:501-10.
3. Holoye PY, et al. (1978) Ann Intern Med 88:47-9.
4. Freeman BA, Crapo JD. (1982) Lab Invest 47:412-26.
5. Sausville EA, et at. (1978) Biochemistry 17:2746-54
6. Kaelin RM, et al (1983) Am Rev Respir Dis 128:132-7
7. Wesselius LJ, Catanzaro A, Wasserman SI. (1984) Am Rev Respir Dis 129:485-90.
8. Moseley PL, et al. (1984) Am Rev Respir Dis 180:1082-6.
9. Katzenstein A, Bloor C, Liebow A (1976) Amer J Pathol 85:210-20.
10. Lindenschmidt RC, et al. (1986). Tox Applied Pharm 85:69-77.
11. Lazo, JS and Pham, ET. (1984) J Pharmacol Exp Ther 228:13-18.
12. Shami SG and Evans MJ. (1986). Exp Mol Path 44:344-9.
13. Goldiner PL, et al. (1978) Br Med J 1:1664-7.
14. Tryka AF, et al (1982) Am Rev Respir Dis 126:1074-79.
15. Goad MEP, Tryka AF, Witschi H. (in press). Tox Applied Pharm.
16. Tryka AF, Godleski JJ, Brain JD. (1984) Cancer Treat Rep 68:759-64.
17. Carrington CB, et al (1978) N Engl J Med 801-9.
18. Tryka AF, Witschi H, Lindenschmidt RC. (1985) Exp Mol Pathol 43:348-58.
19. Tryka AF, et al (1983) Exp Lung Res 5:155-70.
20. Brody AR, et al (1981) Exp Lung Res 2:107-20.

Immunoregulation of Growth Factor Release in Bleomycin Induced Lung Disease
J. Kelley, M. Absher, and E.J. Kovacs

INTRODUCTION

Chronic bleomycin-induced pulmonary toxicity results from direct cellular injury followed by aberrant repair and fibrosis. In the wake of the lung injury events induced by bleomycin, alveolar and interstitial macrophages of the lung release immunoregulatory and anabolic cytokines (1). These peptide growth factors (GFs) play an important role in the induction of cellular proliferation and subsequent remodelling of the lung.

The notion that macrophages modulate metabolism of the mesenchyme has its historic origins in the work of Alexis Carrel who observed that granulocytes contained substances capable of inducing fibroblasts to replicate (2). During the past decade our understanding of normal and abnormal cellular growth regulation has rapidly expanded with the elucidation of the molecular structure, regulation, and function of the peptide GFs. These substances resemble circulating endocrine peptide hormones in many respects. However, they differ importantly from the endocrine hormones in that they act over very short distances within the tissue in which they are elaborated. The growing recognition of the role of GFs in the biology of growth and differentiation and malignant transformation culminated in the awarding of the Nobel Prize to Rita Levi-Montalcini and Stanley Cohen in 1986.

Growth factors act on target cells through their interaction with specific high affinity cell surface receptors (3). This leads to rapid transduction of the signal from the membrane to the appropriate intracellular compartment to elicit a specific set of responses. All cells appear capable of responding to multiple growth factors and also presumably secrete one or more growth substances at some point in their lifespan. Production of GFs is a property of many, possibly all cells. The GFs, while best recognized for their capacity to modulate proliferation, can also affect a variety of other cellular functions including motility, cell shape, contractility, and production of matrix proteins (4).

The manner in which the peptide GFs act has been categorized based on the relationship between the effector cell and the target cell for the GF (5). An autocrine mode of action refers to the presence of specific receptors on the same cell releasing the peptide GF. Cells acting in an autocrine mode are therefore capable of controlling their own proliferation; and experimental evidence suggests that certain malignant and fetal cell lines can indeed act in an autocrine mode. The interaction between T cells and interleukin-2 provides an example of how normal cells can also respond in an autocrine fashion.

In contrast, paracrine secretion involves release of the GF by the responsible effector cell with secondary response by an adjacent target cell. Paracrine secretion appears to be the dominant feature of growth and of remodelling of differentiated tissue. Peptide growth factors can be further subdivided according to the specific point in the G_0/G_1 transition of the cell cycle at which they act (6). Growth factors which are required to initiate the earliest events involved in entry of quiescent cells into the cell cycle are termed "competence" factors, while those that cause the cell to continue to progress through the G_0/G_1 transition have been termed "progression" factors (6). Platelet derived growth factor and somatomedin C provide the binary pair of peptide GFs required to induce proliferation of 3T3 and other cell lines (6).

The growing list of monokines, peptide GFs secreted by monocytes and macrophages, is now known to include among others tumor necrosis factor α (TNF α), transforming growth factor β (TGF β), platelet derived growth factor (PDGF), the fibroblast growth factors (FGFs), and interleukin-1 α and β (IL-1). We and others have used the term macrophage-derived growth factors when studying the general effects of these mediators in unfractionated preparations (1). However, there is probably no longer any justification for the notion of a single biochemically discrete peptide which can be termed macrophage derived growth factor.

The purpose of the studies described here was to define the role of monokines released by alveolar macrophages in the process of pulmonary remodelling induced by toxic doses of bleomycin in a rat model and to define the immunologic mechanisms responsible for their induction.

MATERIALS AND METHODS

Methods have been given in detail elsewhere (1, 7-9). In brief, adult male Fischer 344 rats maintained in a barrier facility were injected once with a single sublethal dose of 0.50-0.65 mg of bleomycin (Blenoxane[R], Bristol Labs, Syracuse, N.Y.) by direct intrapulmonary injection. At various times thereafter animals were sacrificed, lungs excised, and pulmonary cells and epithelial lining fluid harvested by alveolar lavage. Alveolar macrophages were partially purified by adherence to plastic and cultured in serum free medium for 24 hours to allow secretion of GFs. Harvested medium was extensively dialyzed and concentrated by lyophilization before bioassay ("crude peptide GF") or partially purified by column chromatography on DEAE-Sephacel.

Growth factor acitivty was assessed using the assay developed by Pledger and colleagues (6) in which confluent monolayers of mouse BALB/c 3T3 cells or rat lung fibroblasts were used as target cells. Conditions of assay were devised such that optimal amounts of a source of progeression factor (platelet poor plasma) are present but endogenous competence factor activity is entirely depleted. In such an assay system cell proliferation occurs only upon addition of a fresh source of competence factor. Cell proliferation was monitored through uptake of tritiated thymidine 48 hours after stimulation with GF-containing samples. In some studies cell proliferation was quantitated by changes in absolute cell counts or by autoradiography following exposure to tritiated thymidine. Wherever possible, unknown samples were titrated to yield quantitative estimates of half-maximal growth stimulation.

T-cells were collected from the non-adherent alveolar cells obtained by lavage and purified by panning with monoclonal antibodies directed at rat T cell surface markers (W3/25 and OX8, Accurate Chemical and Scientific Corp., Westbury, N.Y.). For analysis of tissue steady state mRNA levels for collagen and fibronectin mRNAs, lungs were flash frozen and pulverized for total RNA extraction (7).

RESULTS

Following direct intratracheal instillation of sublethal doses of bleomycin into the lungs of adult rats, the amount of GF released by cultured alveolar macrophages rises 3- to 4-fold (1). Maximal secretion of GF by alveolar macrophage takes place with cells harvested and cultured for 24 hours 5 to 10 days following induction of bleomycin injury. There is little or no secretion of GFs by resident pulmonary and peritoneal cells in the absence of tissue injury or specific stimulation by lectins. The crude GF released by macrophages harvested from injured lungs has a molecular weight >14 kDa (as determined by dialysis), is heat stable at 56°C for 30 minutes, and can be partially purified by liquid chromatography on DEAE-Sephacel resin. In this regard, it differs from purified platelet derived growth factor which is stable to boiling and is strongly cationic. In spite of obvious biochemical differences from platelet derived growth factor, GFs from alveolar macrophages are remarkably similar in biologic action. Most importantly, both crude and partially purified GFs released by alveolar macrophages act as strict competence factors and have no activity as progression factors. The similarity between platelet derived growth factor and crude GFs produced by alveolar macrophages is also reflected in their comparable abilities to induce increased transcription of the early cell cycle proto-oncogene proteins c-myc and c-fos in 3T3 cells(10).

We next asked whether release of GFs by alveolar macrophages could be detected directly in the lungs of animals with pulmonary bleomycin toxicity. To this end, we compared the time course of appearance of titratable GFs activity in the epithelial lining fluid of the lung with the ability of alveolar macrophages to produce these substances. The epithelial lining fluid harvested by lav-age contains levels of biochemically similar GFs which parallel over time the pattern of secretion by cultured macrophages (9). This observation lends support to the notion of in situ release of GFs during bleomycin toxicity. In contrast, plasma from animals exposed to bleomycin contains no increased levels of competence-inducing activity, and circulating blood monocytes do not spontaneously release detectable amounts of GFs. Taken in combination, these observations indicate that the GFs released in situ are both produced and acting locally.

In spite of their action on fibroblast proliferation, preparations of GFs partially purified by DEAE-Sephacel or heparin-sepharose chromatography do not affect collagen synthesis (11). This is in marked contrast to the known effects of purified TGF-β on collagen and fibronectin biosynthesis and deposition (4) but agrees with our own similarly negative observations with purified human platelet derived growth factor (11). Thus the secretion of GFs by macorphages does not appear to directly modulate the transcriptional changes in mRNA levels for connective tissue proteins which have been documented in this model (7).

The production of GFs represents an indirect response of macrophages to bleomycin, as direct application of bleomycin over a wide range of doses to cultured macrophages in no way stimulates growth factor production (1). This negative observation is in contrast to the finding that direct application of such agents as lectins or endotoxin (1) to macrophages in vitro does induce secretion of GFs.

What then might be the physiologic mechanism responsible for triggering release of GFs by alveolar macrophages during bleomycin-induced fibrogenesis? Specific lymphokines are known to be capable of modulating a number of macrophage functions. We therefore tested the hypothesis that T lymphocytes recruited to the lung during bleomycin toxicity might modulate release of GFs by resident or recruited alveolar macrophages. Indeed, the proportion of total lymphocytes found in alveolar lavage fluid rises dramatically following bleomycin instillation, from undetectable numbers to 23% of the total cells (8). Fractionation of subsets of T cells using immobilization with monoclonal antibodies ("panning") indicated that helper T cells (W3/25+) within the lung promote macrophages to release GFs through the secretion of one or more lymphokines (8). In parallel studies, we observed that recombinant gamma interferon can substitute for the crude lymphokines prepared from pulmonary helper T cells in eliciting secretion of GFs by previously inactive lung macrophages. This control experiment makes it unlikely that contamination of lymphocyte supernatant preparations with endotoxin accounts for the observed results.

DISCUSSION

We have used a model of bleomycin-induced pulmonary injury and fibrosis involving the direct intrapulmonary instillation of a sublethal dose of bleomycin in the rat. Release of peptide growth factors (GFs) from macrophages was monitored by proliferation of already confluent cultures of adult rodent fibroblasts in medium depleted of other competence factors. Within 1-3 days of a single instilled dose of bleomycin the amount of GFs detectable in epithelial lining fluid rose markedly, reaching a maximum at 7-10 days (9). This rise paralleled the amount of growth factors produced per macrophage. The growth factor resembled previously described mediators produced by monocyte cell lines in being a strict competence factor. That is, it required the presence of known progression factors such as somatomedin C but was unable to complement with other known competence factors such as platelet derived growth factor (12). Moreover, alveolar macrophages from normal rat lungs are capable of producing similar growth factors when stimulated in vitro with lipopolysaccharide or lectins (1).

Studies with pulmonary lymphocytes harvested during the course of bleomycin-induced injury indicate that these cells are capable of releasing lymphokines which in turn induce growth factor production by unstimulated alveolar macrophages. These lymphokines by themselves,

however, do not directly stimulate fibroblast replication. Hence these studies underscore the importance of
multicellular interactions in the anabolic phase of
pulmonary remodelling which follows drug induced injury
(Fig 1).

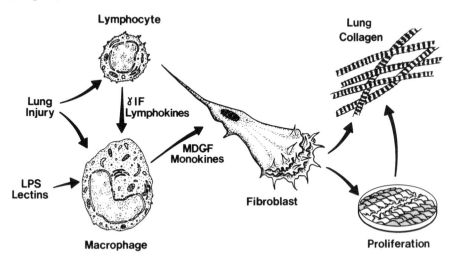

Fig. 1. Schema showing the cytokine cascade involved
in controlling fibroblast proliferation and matrix
production in bleomycin pulmonary toxicity.

Are GFs released within the pulmonary interstitium,
the compartment where mesenchymal remodelling takes
place? There is indirect evidence that this is indeed the
case and that GFs are both released and active in the
interstitium. Bennett and colleagues have recently isolated macrophages from the pulmonary interstitium of
asbestos-exposed rat and have shown that (like their
alveolar counterparts) these cells secreted increased
amounts of GFs when compared to control macrophages (13).
    TGF-β clearly affects collagen and fibronectin
synthesis (4). This finding is at odds with our own
observation that partially purified preparations of GFs
from alveolar macrophages do not appear to affect
collagen synthesis (10). And yet it is clear that there
is marked elevation of collagen synthesis following

bleomycin exposure in the lung and that this is con-
trolled at a translational level (7). Differential
kinetics of expression of cytokines over time as the
lesion develops could explain this discrepancy. Alter-
nately, TGF-β may not be one of the dominant monokines
released by alveolar macrophages in this model.

The observation that during bleomycin-induced
pulmonary toxicity alveolar macrophages release GFs with
a net stimulatory effect for fibroblasts is in accord
with studies of cultured monocyte and macrophage cell
lines (12). However, under certain experimental conditions the observed effects on proliferation can be
altered: studies of human macrophages have been presented
(14) in which the net effect of secreted mediators is
inhibitory rather than stimulatory. This seeming contra-
diction appears to result from several technical factors.
These include the preferred conditions of assay, such as
the presence of whole unfractionated serum, differences
of species, and the nature of the dominant GFs released
by cells in different tissues. It is well recognized that
there are clear differences between the overall effect of
GFs in different species and even from different organs
(15). Failure to remove prostaglandins and other inhibitory low molecular weight molecules by dialysis of crude
macrophage culture medium can also result in inhibition
of target cell growth. Furthermore, the net balance of
anabolic and catabolic cytokines may change over time
during a disease process. Additionally, it is now
recognized that combinations of monokines act differently
from the individual component monokines (16). These
seemingly conflicting observations point emphasize that
peptide GFs interact with each other as well as with a
variety of other biologically active agents in promoting
tissue remodelling. In this model of bleomycin toxicity,
however, it is clear that the net effect of such inter-
acting cytokines is anabolic in nature.

This point has been emphasized through the quantitative analysis of mesenchymal cell populations in the lung following bleomycin administration (17). Using large rats and multiple intratracheal doses of bleomycin, an approach slightly different from the methods described herein, we have shown that there is a 250 percent increase in the number of fibroblasts in the lung two weeks after the initiation of injury. Furthermore, many of the cells have altered morphology and cytoskeletal components suggesting that they have undergone major phenotypic changes.

The efficacy of growth factors in the remodelling process is further emphasized by the fact that fibroblasts cultured from the fibrosing lungs of bleomycin-treated rats exhibit a relative resistance to serum stimulated proliferation (18). The reasons behind this resistance are unclear. Thus the net increase in fibroblast numbers observed in the bleomycin-treated rat lung (17) indicates that locally secreted GFs are capable of overcoming cellular resistance to growth.

In conclusion, these studies of locally secreted GFs have helped us to understand the molecular mechanisms involved in pulmonary remodelling in response to bleomycin induced injury. These investigations point to the importance of multicellular interactions in the anabolic phase of pulmonary remodelling which follows drug induced injury. The recognition of the immunologic mechanisms (e.g. T cell release of lymphokines) controlling GF secretion should provide future directions in the development of strategies of early detection of damage and repair, and ultimately the means of avoiding the irreversible toxic pulmonary manifestations associated with this valuable anticancer agent.

ACKNOWLEDGEMENTS
Dr. James Hildebran, Lynn Chrin, and Ann Hartman contributed to some of the studies described herein. Supported by Vermont Pulmonary SCOR (HL 14212).

REFERENCES

1. Kovacs, E.J., Kelley, J. (1985) J. Leukocyte Biol. 37: 1-14.
2. Carrel, A. (1922) J. Exp. Med. 35: 385-391.
3. Goustin, Leof, E.B., Shipley, G.D., Moses, H.L. (1986) Cancer Res. 46: 1015-1029.
4. Ignotz, R.A., Massague, J. (1986) J. Biol. Chem. 261: 4337-4342.
5. Sporn, M.B., Todaro, G.J. (1980) N. Engl. J. Med. 303: 878-880.
6. Pledger, W.J., Stiles, C.D., Antoniades, H.N., Scher, C.D., (1977) Proc. Natl. Acad. Sci. USA 74: 4481-4490.
7. Kelley, J., Chrin, L., Shull, S., Rowe, D.W., Cutroneo, K.B. (1985) Biochem. Biophys. Res. Comm. 131: 836-843.
8. Kovacs, E.J., Kelley, J. (1985) Am. J. Pathol. 121: 261-268.
9. Kovacs, E.J., Kelley, J. (1986) Am. Rev. Respir. Dis. 133: 68-72.
10. Kovacs, E.J., Hartman, A., Howard, H.A., Kelley, J. (1986) In: Biological Regulation of Cell Proliferation eds. Baserga, R. Foa, P. Metcalf, D. Polli, E.E. (Raven Press, New York), pp. 307-310.
11. Hildebran, J.N., Chrin, L., Kelley, J. (1986) Am. Rev. Respir. Dis. 133: A257.
12. Gillespie, G.Y., Estes, J.E., Pledger, W.J. (1985) In: Lymphokines 11, ed. Pick, E. (Academic Press, Orlando), pp. 213-242.
13. Bennett, R.A., Overby, L.H., Brody, A.R. (1987) Am. Rev. Respir. Dis. 135: A164.
14. Elias, J.A., Rossman, M.D., Zurier, R.B., Daniele, R.P. (1985) Am. Rev. Respir. Dis. 131: 94-99.
15. Shimokado, K., Raines, E.W., Madtes, D.K., Barrett, T.B., Benditt, E.P., Ross, R. (1985) Cell 43: 277-286.
16. Elias, J.A., Gustilo, K., Baeder, W., Freundlich, B. (1987) J. Immunol. 138: 3812-3816.
17. Adler, K.B., Callahan, L.M., Evans, J.N. (1986) Am. Rev. Respir. Dis. 133: 1043-1048.
18. Absher, M., Hildebran, J., Trombley, L., Woodcock-Mitchell, J., Marsh, J. (1984) Am. Rev. Respir. Dis. 129: 125-129.

Pulmonary Toxicity of Anticancer Drugs: Alterations in Endothelial Cell Function
J.D. Catravas

Pulmonary toxicity is a prominent side effect of many anticancer drugs. Although the marrow-sparing antibiotic bleomycin has been identified as the antineoplastic agent with the most serious, life threatening and dose limiting pulmonary toxicity, a number of other drugs have also been reported to produce lung injury; these include carmustine, chlorambucil, cyclophosphamide, cytarabine HCl, estramustine, lomustine, melphalan, methotrexate, mitomycin, procarbazine and semustine[1]. Ionizing radiation, a common adjunct to cancer chemotherapy, is also a powerful pulmonary toxin.

Lung injury after bleomycin and radiation in particular, but with many of the aforementioned drugs as well, most evidently involves the development of interstitial pneumonitis, initially, which can lead to fibrosis. In 1974, Adamson and Bowden observed that endothelial damage was the earliest locus of cellular toxicity after iv bleomycin to mice[2]. This was soon confirmed by others[3]. Within 2-3 days after iv administration of 125 mg bleomycin per kg body weight to mice, endothelial cells were swollen and necrotic (Figure 1-left); this was followed by rapid regeneration during day 5-8 as reflected in increased mitotic index (^{3}H-thymidine uptake; Figure 1-right). Endothelial cell regeneration coincided with type I cell lesions and the beginning of the chronic toxic response[4]. Similar observations were reported after intraperitoneal administration of bleomycin to mice, except for the protraction of the toxicity,

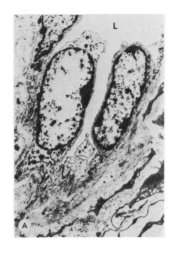
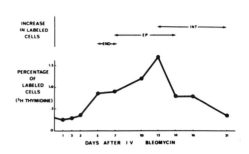

FIGURE 1: Left: Edematous cytoplasm with nuclear lysis in endothelial cells lining the vascular lumen (L) 3 days after iv bleomycin (120 mg/kg; x 5000). Right: Percent ³H-thymidine labelled cells after iv bleomycin (120 mg/kg); cell types showing increased thymidine incorporation were identified by differential counting. END: endothelial; EP: epithelial; INT: interstitial (Reprinted with permission from Ref. 4)

with endothelial lesions appearing approximately two weeks after administration[4].

The effects of bleomycin on normal endothelium can be devastating. In bovine aortic endothelial cell monolayers, two hours exposure to clinically relevant doses of the drug produced endothelial cell retraction and attachment of subsequently added platelets or tumor cells. This was also observed with other antineoplastic agents such as vincristine and BCNU[5]. These studies illustrate that antineoplastic drugs can severely affect both structure and function of pulmonary endothelium, by exposing the basement membrane (loss of barrier function) and promoting adhesion of thrombogenic platelets (thus reversing the normal antithrombotic function of the cell) or tumor cells (promoting metastases). In fact, functional impairment of endothelium by antineoplastic agents is poorly understood. It can occur undetected in the absence of structural damage and may still prove to be an important component of the overall toxicity.

In addition to their antithrombotic properties (presumed to

depend on the release of prostacyclin) pulmonary endothelial cells possess a variety of other functions. In particular, the plasma membrane is equipped with numerous enzymes (angiotensin converting enzyme, 5'-nucleotidase, carbonic anhydrase, lipoprotein lipase), transporters for biogenic compounds (norepinephrine, serotonin, adenosine, prostaglandins) and receptors of pharmacologic (muscarinic, histamine, beta adrenergic) or pathologic (Fc, C3b) importance. In recent years, endothelial cells have also been discovered to participate in the regulation of vascular tone via the production and release of endothelium derived relaxing factors (EDRF) or endothelium derived constricting factors (EDCF).

Functional endothelial impairment after primarily bleomycin has been studied by various investigators. Bleomycin produces variable changes in angiotensin converting enzyme (ACE) activity of lung homogenates from different species. In the rat, a decrease in ACE activity has been observed 3-5 weeks after ip administration[6] as well as a transient decrease up to 10-15 days after intratracheal administration[7] which returned to control levels 2-3 weeks after treatment[7,8]. In the rabbit, lung ACE decreased four weeks after subcutaneous administration of bleomycin[9] but returned to control levels by eleven weeks after treatment[10]. Conversely, no changes were observed 4 weeks after it administration of bleomycin to rabbits[11]. In mice, ip or sc administration of bleomycin resulted in a dose dependent (ip) increase in lung ACE during 6-7 weeks of treatment[12].

Serum angiotensin converting enzyme is a soluble enzyme, immunologically similar to that of lung or kidney and believed to originate from enzyme shedded by either tissue. Serum ACE concentration is approximately 1/50 of the pulmonary endothelial membrane-bound enzyme. Because of the ease in determining serum ACE activity, numerous attempts have been made to correlate serum enzyme levels with various types and degrees of lung injury, most notably sarcoidosis. Changes in serum ACE after bleomycin do not always parallel those in lung ACE. Thus, it

administration of bleomycin causes an increase in serum ACE of rats[7], but not of rabbits[11]. Interestingly, in rabbits, sc administration of bleomycin causes a prolonged reduction in serum ACE[9,10] which is maintained even after lung ACE activity has recovered[10]. In mice, serum ACE levels increase (as do lung) after ip bleomycin[12]. In patients treated for testicular carcinoma, serum ACE activity increased during 126 days of pulsed regimen and in the absence of clinical or radiological evidence of lung damage; serum ACE returned to control levels after cessation of treatment[13].

A different index of endothelial damage by antineoplastic drugs proposes measurements of ACE levels in bronchoalveolar lavage (BAL)[7]. Unlike serum ACE, ACE in BAL has a higher probability of originating from the lung, although not necessarily from the endothelium alone, since other cell types (e.g., macrophages) are known to express the enzyme. After a

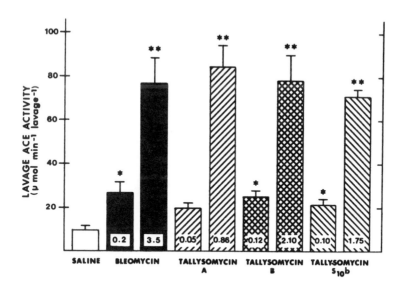

Figure 2. Effect of bleomycin and tallysomycin analogs on the release of ACE into pulmonary lavage fluid. Single it doses (noted within bars as mg/kg) were administered to rats. Animals were lavaged 3 days after dosing. Lavage angiotensin-converting enzyme (ACE) activity data are presented as X±SE of six to eight rats per group. *p< 0.05, **p <0.01 with respect to control. (Reprinted with permission from ref. 14).

single it injection of bleomycin, rats develop a dose-dependent and time dependent increase in BAL ACE[7]. Newman and colleagues[14] have used this procedure to demonstrate equitoxic activity among equitherapeutic doses of bleomycin and tallysomycin A, B or $S_{10}b$ (Fig 2).

In an effort to more directly assess endothelial damage by anticancer drugs, measurements of single pass transpulmonary disposition of substrates for ACE and other endothelial plasmalemmal enzymes or transporters were performed in rabbits and rats. Four weeks after sc treatment with bleomycin, and at doses producing no obvious interstitial changes, transplasmalemmal endothelial removal of serotonin or norepinephrine from the pulmonary circulation of anesthetized rabbits was significantly reduced[15]. These changes, however, were transient and both of these functions had returned to control levels 6 weeks after termination of treatment. At that time, transpulmonary metabolism of Benzoyl-Phe-Ala-Pro (BPAP; a specific substrate of endothelial membrane-bound ACE) had not changed either. Utilizing similar techniques, the functional integrity of pulmonary endothelium was studied following it bleomycin to rabbits. In this model, a dose-dependent decrease in serotonin and norepinephrine removal and BPAP metabolism were observed 4 weeks after treatment (Fig 3). Whereas changes in norepinephrine removal and BPAP metabolism coincided with increased collagen deposition, serotonin removal was impaired at a subfibrotic dose, suggesting increased sensitivity of the serotonin transporter to the toxic actions of bleomycin, a finding in agreement with other models of pulmonary toxicity (e.g., microembolization).

Utilizing a similar approach, serotonin transport and BPAP metabolism were impaired 2 weeks after a single intratracheal injection of 7.5 U BLM/kg to rats (Fig. 4). In these studies, the animals were sacrificed and the lungs were perfused in situ

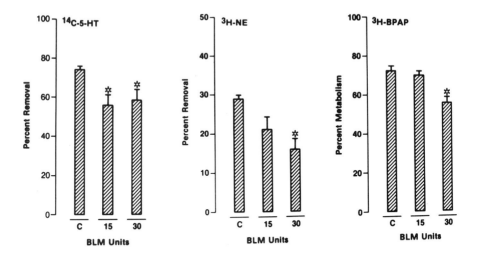

Figure 3. Single pass transpulmonary removal of ^{14}C-5-hydroxytryptamine, ^{3}H-norepinephrine or transpulmonary metabolism of the ACE substrate ^{3}H-BPAP, in vivo, in rabbits treated with a single intratracheal injection of saline (C) or 15 units (6 U/kg) or 30 units (11 U/kg) bleomycin. Measurements were made 4 weeks after treatment and represent measures ± 1 SE *p < 0.05 from C. (N=4 per measurement. Reprinted with permission from ref. 15)

with an albumin containing physiologic salt, blood-free solution at constant inflow pressure. Significant increases in lung hydroxyproline levels were observed at this but not at a lower dose (1.7 U/kg) of bleomycin[8].

Another important property of lung, and of endothelium in particular, involves prostaglandin synthesis from membrane phospholipids. Intratracheal administration of bleomycin to hamsters produced a transient, initial (4-14 days) increase in

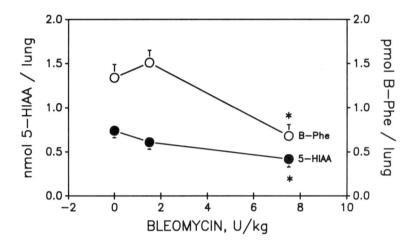

Figure 4. Effects of a sub-fibrotic and a fibrotic dose of bleomycin (2 weeks after it administration) on serotonin accumulation in lung (expressed as nmol of product, 5-hydroxyindole acetic acid or 5-HIAA) and BPAP (ACE substrate) conversion in the pulmonary circulation (expressed as pmol of the product benzoyl-Phe) in rats whose lungs were perfused in situ with a blood-free Krebs-albumin (5%) solution at 20 cmH_2O inflow pressure. N=11 (0 dose), 6 (1.7 /kg) or 11 (7.5 /kg). Means ± SE *p < 0.05 compared the 0 dose (saline) group.

plasma thromboxane B_2 and 6-keto-prostaglandin $F_{1\alpha}$ levels (stable products of thromboxane A_2 and prostacyclin, respectively)[16]. Since prostaglandins are not stored, but depend on release of membrane-associated arachidonic acid, these studies suggest an early interaction of bleomycin with the cell membrane.

While the aforementioned studies suggest endothelial dysfunction following administration of antineoplastic drugs, they do not exclude the possibility for alternative explanations.

For example, we reported on the amounts of serotonin or norepinephrine transported, but not on the transporter itself. Thus the observed changes could be due, at least in part, to altered time of interaction between the substrate and the transporter. Similarly, plasma levels of thromboxane were measured but not thromboxane synthetase or cyclo-oxygenase. In an effort to study the enzyme or transporter directly, but still maintain the advantage of the in vivo model and the assurance of examining an endothelial process, we have recently applied new methodology[17] to measure Michaelis-Menten enzyme kinetic constants during suspected endothelial dysfunction.

Irradiation of the chest (30 Gy) produced elevations in the apparent Km values of two endothelial plasmalemmal enzymes: ACE (for BPAP) and 5'-nucleotidase (for 5'-AMP) at 2, 24 and 48 hrs post injury[18]. The experimental values were significantly higher from both pre-irradiation levels within the same group and corresponding levels in the sham-irradiated group (Fig. 5) and suggest a decreased affinity of the substrates for the enzymes. Since the two enzymes have strikingly different substrate requirements, these findings point towards a more generalized effect of radiation on the plasma membrane. Similar studies are currently underway with antineoplastic drugs.

This chapter has outlined a number of changes in pulmonary endothelial function which occur during the early phases of bleomycin-induced lung injury. Additional functional alterations will probably be revealed in the near future. Still, there are two issues that must be addressed in order to properly understand these observations. First, it remains to be shown whether changes in endothelial function in response to bleomycin (or other anticancer drugs) are a result of drug-induced endothelial toxicity rather than a concurring drug-enzyme interaction. For example, Lazo et al. have demonstrated that bleomycin-induced inhibition of ACE activity in cultured endothelial cell marolayers is due to bleomycin chelation of Zn^{+2} in the ACE molecule (Zn^{+2} is necessary for ACE

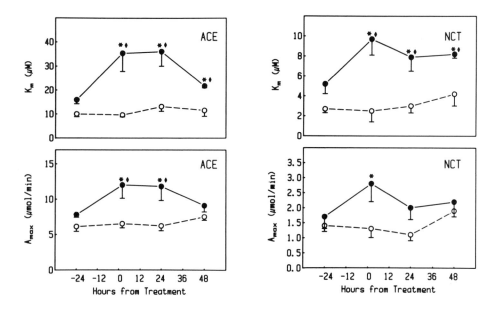

Figure 5: Apparent Michaelis-Menten, constants of endothelial bound 5'-nucleotidase for 5'-AMP and ACE for BPAP measured in conscious rabbits exposed to 3000 rad radiation to the chest (open circles: shave radiated controls; closed circles: experimental). Mean ± 1 SE of 4 controls and 6 radiated rabbits. *p <0.05 compared to the control value within each group. **:p< 0.05 between same time values of the control and irradiated groups. (Reprinted from ref. 18)

activity) and can be reversed or prevented by the addition of Zn^{+2} or other divalent cations[19]. Whether a similar mechanism exists in vivo, remains to be seen. Secondly, the contribution of endothelial injury (structural or functional) to the pathogenesis of the chronic lesion (fibrosis) after bleomycin and other drugs is still unclear. Possible theories for such contribution have been advanced, such as a) easier access of the drug to the interstitium when the endothelium is injured[20] and b) the existence of endothelium-derived fibroblast proliferating factors[21].

ACKNOWLEDGEMENTS

Acknowledgement is given to Jacki McKnight for her expert preparation of this manuscript. Part of this work was supported by HL 31422, the American Lung Association of Georgia, the American Heart Association of Georgia and the American Cancer Society. J. Catravas is an Established Investigator of the American Heart Association.

REFERENCES

1. The Medical Letter 29:29-36 (1987)
2. Adamson, IYR and Bowden, DH. (1974) Amer. J. Pathol. 77:185-198.
3. Aso, Y., Yoneda, K. and Kikkawa, Y. (1976) Lab Invest. 35:558.
4. Adamson, IYR and Bowden, DH. (1979) Amer. J. Pathol. 96:531-538.
5. Nicolson, GL and Custead, SE. (1985) Canc. Res. 45:331-336.
6. Tom, WM and Montgomery, MR. (1980) Toxicol. Appl. Pharmacol. 53:64-74.
7. Newman, RA, Kimberly, PJ, Stweart, JA and Kelley, J. (1980) Canc. Res. 40:3621-3626.
8. Catravas, JD, Watkins, CA and Newman, RA. (1987) Amer. Rev. Resp. Dis. 135:A257.
9. Lazo, JS, Catravas, JD and Gillis, CN. (1981) Biochem. Pharmacol. 30:2577-2584.
10. Lazo, JS, Catravas, JD, Dobuler, KJ and Gillis, CN. (1983) Toxicol. Appl. Pharmacol. 69:276-282.
11. Catravas, JD, Lazo, JS, Dobuler, KD, Mills, LR and Gillis, CN. (1983) Amer. Rev. Resp. Dis. 128:740-746.
12. Lazo, JS. (1981) Toxicol. Appl. Pharmacol. 59:395-404.
13. Sorensen, PG, Romer, FK and Cortes, S. (1984) Eur. J. Canc. Clin. Oncol. 20:1405-1408.
14. Newman, RA, Hacker, MP, Kimberly, PJ and Braddock, JM. (1981) Toxicol. Appl. Pharmacol. 61:469-474.
15. Catravas, JD, Lazo, JS and Gillis, CN. (1981) J. Pharmacol Exp. Ther. 217:524-529.
16. Chandler, DB and Giri, SN. (1983) Amer. Rev. Resp. Dis. 128:71-76.
17. Catravas, JD. (1986) Adv. Exp. Med. 198:445-451.
18. Catravas, JD and Burch, SE. (1987) Toxicol Appl. Pharmacol.
19. Lazo, JS, Lynch, TJ and McCallister, J. (1983) Amer. Rev. Resp. Dis. 134:73-78.
20. Lazo, JS. (1986) Biochem. Pharmacol. 35:1919-1923.
21. Adamson, IYR and Bowden, DA. (1983) Amer. J. Pathol. 112:274.

Pulmonary Metabolic Inactivation of Bleomycin and Protection from Drug-Induced Lung Injury
J.S. Lazo, J.E. Mignano, and S.M. Sebti

INTRODUCTION

Many conventional antineoplastic agents and investigational biological response modifiers produce pulmonary injury. The pulmonary fibrosis associated with the glycopeptide-like antibiotics of the bleomycin class is, however, one of the most life-threatening. This untoward effect is characterized by an increased pulmonary content of fibronectin, glycosaminoglycans, and collagen, especially type III relative to type I collagen. It is generally assumed that bleomycin-induced pulmonary fibrosis is caused by a bleomycin-iron-oxygen ternary complex, which results either in cleavage of genomic DNA or lipid peroxidation (1, 2). In this manuscript we will focus upon one major biochemical factor responsible for the preferential damage to the lungs: the lack of a protective enzyme called bleomycin hydrolase.

BLEOMYCIN METABOLISM IN VIVO

The propensity of bleomycin to produce pulmonary fibrosis was identified both preclinically and clinically soon after the drug was discovered (3, 4). Umezawa et al. (5) examined the organ distribution of bleomycin in an attempt to determine if the selective injury was related to preferential pulmonary drug uptake. Radioactivity was found in all organs with no apparent selective uptake in the lungs. Similar data were obtained by Lazo and Humphreys (6) using the most common component of the clinical mixture, bleomycin A_2, which was radiolabeled. When Umezawa and co-workers examined the biological activity of different organs containing the radioactive bleomycin using a growth inhibition assay with <u>Bacillus</u> <u>subtilis</u> (5), they found considerable discrepancy. In particular, lungs and skin were found to have a much higher biological activity per unit of bleomycin derived radioactivity compared to organs such as livers kidneys or spleens. These data suggested the possibility of bleomycin metabolism. Because the bioassay used by Umezawa et al. (5) to evaluate bleomycin content could have been influenced by a variety of components in the organ homogenates (6,7), Lazo and co-workers (6) developed a high-pressure liquid chromatography (hplc) system that allowed them to demonstrate unequivocally that metabolites of bleomycin A_2 were formed <u>in</u> <u>vivo</u>. Almost half of the radioactivity found in the kidneys, liver, and spleen of C57BL/6 mice was metabolized 1 hour after a subcutaneous drug injection; little metabolite formation was seen in pulmonary tissue (Fig. 1). When lungs were examined 12 to 24 hr after either an intratracheal or subcutaneous injection of $[^3H]$ bleomycin A_2, significant quantities of metabolites were detected (8). Thus, based upon hplc analysis of organ homogenates, multiple metabolites may exist. The most prominent metabolite seen in liver and kidneys 0.5 to 2 hr after injection of $[^3H]$ bleomycin A_2 comigrates on hplc with a form of bleomycin A_2 that is deamidated in the beta-aminoalanine moiety and is discussed below.

BLEOMYCIN METABOLISM IN VITRO

The apparent loss of bleomycin antibacterial activity in organ homogenates after i.p. injection of radiolabeled bleomycin in mice led Umezawa and co-workers

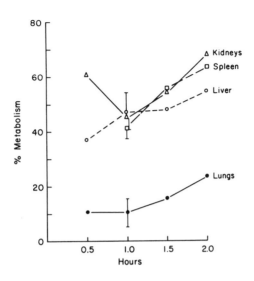

Figure 1. Metabolism of [³H]Bleomycin A₂ In Vivo. The percentage of the total radioactivity that was not [³H]Bleomycin A₂ was calculated in organs at various times by hplc. (Reproduced from Ref. 6).

(5) to examine the metabolic fate of this drug in vitro. In seminal work, they identified an enzyme activity in the postmicrosomal supernatant fraction that inactivated bleomycin. The relative levels of inactivating activity varied among organs but generally was lowest in lung and skin homogenates. Subsequent hplc studies by Yoshioka et al. (9) and Lazo et al. (6, 10) indicated that the inactivation was due to the formation of a single metabolite thought to be generated by the hydrolysis of the carboxyamide moiety in the beta-aminoalanine portion of the bleomycin molecule. The chemical nature of the metabolite (called deamido bleomycin) was deduced based upon: (a) a stoichiometric release of one mole of ammonia per mole of bleomycin metabolized, (b) comparison of the chemical composition of acid hydrolysis products formed

with unmetabolized bleomycin and deamido bleomycin and, (c) a shift in the pK_a of the alpha amino group of the beta aminoalanine moiety from 7.4 to 9.4 (1, 11). Due to the pK_a change, it is believed that at physiological pH the free-carboxylic acid of the aminoalanine moiety rather than the protonated alpha amino group occupies the fifth coordination site of the bleomycin-iron-oxygen ternany complex. This leads to a marked decrease in the formation of an "activated" bleomycin complex competent in performing radical chemistry (12, 13). The deamidated bleomycin is 1/100th as potent as the parent compound in degrading DNA (14) and at inhibiting bacterial or tumor growth (1, 11). In addition, the deamido bleomycin product lacks the ability to produce pulmonary fibrosis in laboratory animals (6).

The sensitivity of pulmonary tissue to bleomycin is inversely proportional to the levels of bleomycin hydrolase activity as measured in vitro. Lung homogenates from species, such as rabbits, which are known to be resistant to bleomycin-induced fibrosis, have significantly higher levels of bleomycin hydrolase than species, such as mice, which are relatively sensitive to bleomycin (6). Moreover, inbred murine strains also display differences in sensitivity to bleomycin-induced pulmonary fibrosis (i.e. C57Bl/6 > DBA > BALB/c) (15, 16) and this difference is inversely related to the pulmonary levels of bleomycin hydrolase (17). No significant differences in kidney or hepatic bleomycin hydrolase have been noted in these strains. Thus, high levels of this inactivating enzyme appear to protect lungs and other organs against bleomycin-induced toxicity. It has also been proposed that elevated levels of bleomycin hydrolase engender a bleomycin-resistant phenotype to malignant cells and that the enzyme is dominantly expressed in somatic cell hybrids (18).

PULMONARY CELLULAR LOCATION OF BLEOMYCIN HYDROLASE

Results from Lazo et al. (19) indicate that bleomycin hydrolase is heterogeneously localized in pulmonary cells. Using freshly isolated and cultured cells, they found high levels of enzyme activity in rabbit pulmonary endothelial cells, fibroblasts, and alveolar macrophages and undetectable levels in type II epithelial cells. Since type II epithelial cells may be stem cells for the formation of type I cells, the low levels of bleomycin hydrolase activity in type II epithelial cells may explain the findings of Adamson and Bowden (20) that epithelial type I cells were extremely sensitive to bleomycin toxicity. It has been proposed (19) that the pulmonary toxicity of bleomycin may be related to an initial adverse effect on either epithelial or endothelial cells lacking bleomycin hydrolase activity. The development of an antibody to bleomycin hydrolase (21) should be very useful in mapping the precise cellular localization of this protective enzyme in pulmonary tissue and testing this hypothesis.

CHARACTERISTICS OF BLEOMYCIN HYDROLASE

Previous attempts to characterize the biochemical properties of bleomycin hydrolase have been thwarted by the instability of the enzyme and difficulties in its purification. Umezawa et al. (22) initially examined the enzyme in a partially purified form (27-fold). They found that the enzyme had some properties, which were similar to those of hepatic aminopeptidases, but could be partially separated by gel filtration from a majority of the aminopeptidase B-like activity in liver preparations. Sebti and Lazo (23) utilized fast protein liquid chromatography to demonstrate unequivocally that bleomycin hydrolase was distinct from all detectable pulmonary aminopeptidases (Fig. 2).

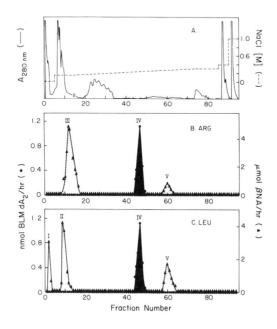

Figure 2. Anion-exchange Mono Q chromatography of rabbit lung cytosol. An aliquot of the 105,000g supernatant was loaded onto the Mono Q column and eluted with various NaCl gradients in 10mM Tris (pH 7.4) buffer as described in Reference 23. Absorbance at 280 nm (solid line) was monitored and is shown with the NaCl gradient profile (dashed line) in panel A. The full scale at 280nm was 2 absorbance units for the first 15 fractions of the profile and 0.5 absorbance unit for the remaining of the profile. BLM hydrolase (closed circles, blackened area) and aminopeptidase B (panel B) and aminopeptidase N (panel C) (closed triangles, hatched area) were assayed as described in Reference 23.

In addition to charge characteristics, bleomycin hydrolase was distinguishable from aminopeptidase B based upon its enzymatic stability, molecular mass, and sensitivity to inhibitors and activators (23). Using sequential anion exchange, hydrophobic attraction, and affinity chromatography, Sebti, et al., (24) have successfully purified bleomycin hydrolase to homogeneity from rabbit lungs. The 6000-fold purified enzyme exhibited a molecular mass of 250 kDa on nondenaturing PAGE and gel filtration chromatography and a single band of 50 kDa on SDS-PAGE. These results suggest the enzyme normally exists in a pentameric form. Moreover, bleomycin hydrolase activity was inhibited by NEM suggesting that it is a thiol enzyme (Table 1). Bleomycin hydrolase interacts with regions of the bleomycin molecule that are far removed from the site of metabolism. Alterations in the terminal amine and the carbohydrate moieties greatly affect the Km and the Vmax, respectively (25). A summary of the relevant biochemical features of rabbit pulmonary bleomycin hydrolase are seen in Table 1.

Recently, Nishimura et al. (21) developed a hybridoma clone that produces an IgM monoclonal antibody to bleomycin hydrolase. An immunoaffinity column was prepared with this antibody and used to purify (1300-fold) rabbit liver bleomycin hydrolase. Analysis of the native form of the rabbit liver enzyme by these authors suggested that the subunits were 48kDa and the native enzyme had a slightly larger mass (ca. 300 kDa) than that of the lung enzyme found by Sebti et al. (24) (Table 1). Additionally, a hexameric enzyme was proposed (21). It is not yet certain whether the slight differences in molecular mass between rabbit lung and liver enzyme exist or whether the assigned mass values reflect differences in preparations or analytical procedures. Nonetheless, both enzyme preparations showed similar inhibitor profiles and

Table 1

CHARACTERISTICS OF RABBIT PULMONARY
AND LIVER BLEOMYCIN HYDROLASE[a]

	Pulmonary	Liver
Cellular Location	cytoplasmic	cytoplasmic
Molecular Mass	250 kDa (native)	300 kDa
	50 kDa (denatured)	48 kDa
$t1/2$ (56°C)	25 min	−
(37°C)	10 hr	−
(4°C)	5 days	3 days
pH Optimum	7.0 to 7.5	6.8 to 7.8
pI	5.3, 4.5, and 4.3	5.2
Amino Acid Composition	48% hydrophobic and 37% acidic	−
K_m (mM)	1.3 (BLM A_2)	0.79 (BLM B_2)
Vmax (umoles/mg (protein x hr)	5.6 (BLM A_2)	380 (BLM B_2)
Inhibitors	leupeptin	leupeptin
	N-ethylameimide	N-ethylaneimide
	TLCK	TLCK
	puromycin	
	divalent cations	divalent cations
	TH-RH	IE-64
	Substance P	

[a] Data for pulmonary enzyme from Sebti et al. (24) and for liver from Nishimura et al. (21).

kinetic properties. The use of a monoclonal antibody by Nishimura et al. (21) may have selected for only one of the isoforms of bleomycin hydrolase, since the liver enzyme isolated with the antibody exhibited only one pI (i.e. 5.2). The monoclonal antibody apparently recognizes only a subset of bleomycin hydrolases, since the antibody failed to immunoprecipitate bleomycin hydrolase from MH134 and Ehrlich ascites carcinoma cells.

The availability of purified bleomycin hydrolase has permitted our laboratory to study further the biochemical and molecular characteristics of the enzyme. Rabbit pulmonary bleomycin hydrolase was found to have a blocked amino terminus that prevented N-terminal sequence analysis. Thus, we digested bleomycin hydrolase with trypsin and generated more than 50 detectable peaks on hplc. One major peak was isolated, sequenced and found to contain 25 amino acids. This amino acid sequence has been employed to construct a 36-mer oligonucleotide using the method of Lathe (26). The 36-mer hybridizes to a single band of 1.8 kb by Northern blot analysis with rabbit liver, spleen, and lung mRNA. In addition, this 36-mer also hybridized with a 1.8 kb mRNA species from HL-60 human promyleocytic leukemia cells and from the liver and kidneys of baboon, chicken, and bullfrog. Therefore, bleomycin hydrolase appears not only to be widely distributed among cells in a given organ (8) but also among organs of different species.

Recent work in our laboratory has focused upon elucidating the complete amino acid and gene sequence of rabbit bleomycin hydrolase. To this end, a lambda gt11 rabbit liver cDNA library (gift of Dr. R. Tukey, University of California at San Diego) has been screened using the 36-mer oligonucleotide as a probe. Approximately 750,000 plaques were screened to yield one positive clone. This clone contained a 500 bp Eco RI insert that hybridized strongly with the probe. This insert has been subcloned into a M13 cloning/sequencing vector and is in the process of being sequenced. As the bleomycin hydrolase gene is apparently considerably larger than the recovered 500 bp fragment, the cDNA library is now being rescreened to obtain overlapping or full-length clones of the bleomycin hydrolase gene for sequencing. Once the sequence of the gene is known, it will be compared to known sequences in an attempt to determine the protein family to which the enzyme belongs and also the identity of its normal substrate.

CONCLUSION

Bleomycin hydrolase is a cytosolic thiol containing enzyme of considerable mass (250 to 300kDa) that probably comprises 5 to 6 subunits. In vivo and in vitro studies suggest pulmonary bleomycin hydrolases is extremely important in protecting against bleomycin-induced lung injury. This drug inactivating enzyme is found heterogenously distributed in the cells of the lung and the cellular localization may also be important in determining the extent of lung injury. Furthermore, hybridization studies with an oligonucleotide probe revealed that the enzyme mRNA is widely distributed among species. This suggests that bleomycin hydrolase is highly conserved and could have another important cellular function.

REFERENCES

1. Lazo, J.S., Sebti, S.M. and Filderman. A.E. (1987) Metabolism and Mechanism of Action of Anticancer Drugs. eds. Prough, R.A. and Powis, G. pp. 194-210. (Taylor and Francis, Ltd., London).

2. Ekimoto, H., Takahashi, K., Mutsuda, A., Takita, T., and Umezawa, H. (1985) J. Antibiotics (Tokyo) 38: 1077-1082.

3. Ishizuka, M., Takayama, H., Takeachi, T., and Umezawa, H. (1967) J. Antibiotics (Tokyo) 20: 15-24.

4. Luna, M.A., Bedrossian, C.W.M., Lichtiger, B. and Salem, P.A. (1972) Am. J. Clin. Pathol. 58: 501-510.

5. Umezawa, H., Takeuchi, T., Hori, S., Sawa, T., and Ishizuka, M. (1972) J. Antibiotics (Tokyo) 25: 409-420.

6. Lazo, J.S., and Humphreys, C.J. (1983) Proc. Natl. Acad. Sci., USA, 80: 3064-3068.

7. Thomas, A.H., Newland, P., and Sharma, N.R. (1984) J. Chromatog. 291: 219-230.

8. Lazo, J.S., and Pham, E.T. (1984) J. Pharmacol. Exp. Ther. 228: 13-18.

9. Yoshioka, O., Amano, N., Takahashi, K., Matsuda, A., and Umezawa, H. (1978) In Bleomycin: Current Status and New Developments. eds. Carter, S.K., Crooke, S.T., and Umezawa, H. pp. 35-56. (Academic Press, New York).

10. Lazo, J.S., Boland, C.J., and Schwartz, P.E. (1982) Cancer Res. 42: 4026-4031.

11. Umezawa, H. (1979) In Bleomycin: Chemical, Biochemical, and Biological Aspects. ed. Hecht, S.M. pp. 24-36 (Springer-Verlag, New York).

12. Burger, R.M., Horwitz, S.B., and Peisach, J. (1985) Biochemistry. 24: 3623-3629.

13. Takahashi, K., Ekimoti, H., Aoyagi, S., Koyu, A., Kuramochi, H., Yoshioka, O., Matsuda, A., Fujii, A. and Umezawa, M. (1979) J. Antibiotics (Tokyo) 32: 36-42.

14. Sugiura, Y. (1980) J. Am. Chem. Soc. 102: 5208-5215.

15. Schrier, D.J., Kunkel, R.G. and Pham, S.H. (1983) Am. Rev. Resp. Dis. 127: 63-66.

16. Harrison, J.H. and Lazo, J.S. (1987) Fed. Proc. 46: 1150.

17. Filderman, A.E. and Lazo, J.S. (1986) Am. Rev. Resp. Dis. 133: A72.

18. Akiyama, S.I. and Kuwano, M. (1981) J. Cell. Physiology 107: 147-152.

19. Lazo, J.S., Merrill, W.W., Pham, E.T., Lynch, T.J., McCallister, J.D., and Ingbar, D.H. (1984) J. Pharmacol. Exp. Ther. 231: 583-588.

20. Adamson, I.Y.R. and Bowden, D. (1979) Am. J. Path. 96: 531-538.

21. Nishimura, C., Tanaka, N., Suzuki, H., and Tanaka, N. (1987) Biochemistry 26: 1574-1578.

22. Umezawa, H., Hori, S., Tsutomu, S., Yorhioka, T. and Takeuhi, T. (1974) J. Antibiotics (Tokyo) 27: 419-424.

23. Sebti, S.M. and Lazo, J.S. (1987) Biochemistry 26: 432-437.

24. Sebti, S.M., DeLeon, J.C. and Lazo, J.S. (1987) Biochemistry (In Press; June 1987).

25. Sebti, S.M., DeLeon, J.C., Hecht, S.M. and Lazo, J.S. (1987) Proc. Amer. Assoc. Cancer Res. 28: 17.

26. Lathe, R. (1985) J. Mol. Biol. 183: 1-12.

Biochemical and Molecular Bases of Bleomycin-Induced Pulmonary Fibrosis: Glucocorticoid Intervention
K.R. Cutroneo, D. Cockayne, and K.M. Sterling, Jr.

Bleomycin, a glycopeptide antineoplastic agent, is used to treat several types of malignancies including squamous cell carcinoma of the head and neck, lymphomas and testicular carcinomas (1). Although the mechanism of action of bleomycin is not fully understood, this chemotherapeutic agent does cause DNA damage (2-4) and inhibits DNA synthesis (5, 6). Interaction of bleomycin with purified DNA results in single and double stranded DNA breaks in addition to releasing free bases (2, 7-9). There is also preferential sensitivity of actively transcribing genes in active chromatin to bleomycin (10).

The major and limiting toxicity of bleomycin is pulmonary fibrosis (11-14). Recently, it has been shown that mouse lung lacks detectable bleomycin hydrolase activity, which may determine the fibrogenic properties of bleomycin in lung (15). Collagen content of the lung increases in animals given bleomycin (16-20). A single intratracheal injection of bleomycin results in increases of prolyl hydroxylase activity, soluble protein and proteinaceous hydroxyproline (20). Zapol et al. reported increased collagen content in human lungs of patients

*Supported by NIH Grants HL 31500 and AR 19808
**K. M. Sterling is a Charles H. Revson Fellow.

with pulmonary fibrosis (21). The bleomycin-induced increase of lung collagen content in animals is associated with increased collagen synthesis (22-25). In addition, to changes in collagen metabolism, lung glycosaminoglycan synthesis (26) and lung elastin content (27) are increased.

Corticosteroids have been used to prevent the elevation of proteinaceous hydroxyproline in rats treated with bleomycin. Rats received either 4 or 8 mg/kg, i.p. of triamcinolone on alternate days. Triamcinolone treatment at 4 mg/kg partially blocked the increases of prolyl hydroxylase activity, soluble protein and proteinaceous hydroxyproline. However, triamcinolone at 8 mg/kg completely blocked the elevations of the fibrogenic parameters in bleomycin-treated rats.

Little is known about the molecular mechanism(s) of the regulation of procollagen synthesis by bleomycin. We, as well as others, studied the direct effect of bleomycin on collagen metabolism in IMR-90 human embryonic lung fibroblasts (28, 29). These studies demonstrated that bleomycin increased total collagen synthesis per cell. In addition, Clark et al. (29) found an increase in the ratio of type I to type III collagen in bleomycin-treated IMR-90 human lung fibroblasts.

Bleomycin-induced lung fibrosis involves the participation of many cell types, cell-cell interactions, soluble factors, various biochemical, immunological and morphological changes as well as genetically-induced predisposition. The lung contains many cell types which are affected during the initiation and progression of fibrotic lung disease. Of particular importance is the participation of the alveolar macrophage through its production of protein factor(s) which alters fibroblast growth and regulates collagen production (30-34). The significance of this macrophage-derived factor(s) was appreciated with the demonstration of similar factor(s) in lung explants of bleomycin-treated animals (35).

We will focus mainly on the direct effect of bleomycin on Type I collagen synthesis in fibroblasts, since ninety percent of the collagen produced by fibroblasts is Type I. Type I collagen is also the predominant collagen type increased in bleomycin-induced pulmonary fibrosis and in bleomycin-treated IMR-90 human embryonic lung fibroblasts (29). Bleomycin has direct effects on collagen metabolism of fibroblasts in the lung. There are many similar biochemical changes of collagen metabolism in lung after administration of bleomycin and in fibroblast cultures after the addition of this chemotherapeutic agent. These similarities are as follows: (1) collagen synthesis is increased in lung and in fibroblast cell culture after bleomycin treatment, (2) the onset of increased collagen synthesis in lung is 2-3 days and in fibroblasts is 2 days following bleomycin administration, (3) the dose of bleomycin which increases collagen synthesis _in vivo_ is 25 pg/fibroblast and in cultured fibroblasts is 6 pg/fibroblast, (4) prolyl hydroxylase is increased in lung and in fibroblast culture following bleomycin administration, (5) the ratio of Type I to Type III collagen is increased in fibrotic lung and in bleomycin-treated fibroblasts and (6) collagen degradation is increased in bleomycin-induced fibrotic lung and is also increased in bleomycin-treated lung fibroblasts. The fibroblast thus offers a model system to determine the biochemical and molecular mechanism(s) by which bleomycin increases collagen synthesis and degradation. The development of this _in vitro_ model of the changes in collagen synthesis which take place during the initiation and progression of pulmonary fibrosis also provides a system for screening bleomycin and its analogues for their ability to increase collagen synthesis. These studies may result not only in the elucidation of a molecular basis for bleomycin-induced lung fibrosis, but more importantly, a general mechanism by which other substances induce an accumulation of collagen in fibrotic lung.

One of the most conspicuous effects of bleomycin on fibroblasts is the inhibition of cell growth (28). Bleomycin as low as 0.006 µg/ml inhibited growth of IMR90 human embryonic lung fibroblasts. Total inhibition of cell growth occurred at 3.0 µg/ml. At all doses tested the viability of the cells was ninety percent. In these same cells bleomycin at 3 µg/ml increased collagen synthesis without an effect on noncollagen protein synthesis. Besides stimulating collagen synthesis bleomycin treatment resulted in a three fold increase of prolyl hydroxylase activity. To ensure that bleomycin did not alter the specific activity of the prolyl-t-RNA precursor pool, polysomes were isolated from control and bleomycin treated cells and translated in the wheat germ lysate system. Polysomes isolated from bleomycin-treated cells synthesized more collagen than control polysomes. This stimulatory effect of bleomycin on collagen synthesis is not confined to human embryonic fibroblasts. As seen in Figure 1 this antineoplastic drug specifically increases collagen synthesis in embryonic chick skin and chick lung fibroblasts and in adult rat skin and rat lung fibroblasts. This stimulation of collagen synthesis by bleomycin has also been demonstrated in other fibroblasts. However, in these cells the growth inhibitory effect may also accompany the stimulatory effect of this drug on collagen synthesis.

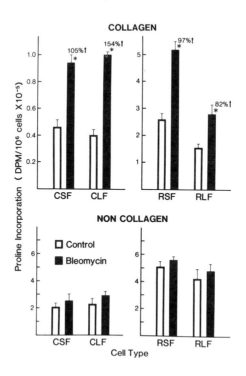

Figure 1: Bleomycin-induced increase of collagen synthesis in various cell types. Chick skin, chick lung, rat
skin and rat lung fibroblasts were grown to late log
phase. The cells were treated with bleomycin for 48 hr.
Two hours before collecting the cells [³H] proline was
added to the media. Collagen and noncollagen protein
synthesis was determined by the collagenase assay. The
values represent the mean ± S.E. of 3-5 cultures.

In an attempt to define the molecular mechanism by
which bleomycin increases collagen synthesis in cultured
fibroblasts, embryonic chick skin and lung fibroblasts
were treated with bleomycin and total cellular Type I

procollagen mRNAs were determined by dot blot hybridization (Figure 2). Bleomycin treatment did not alter the total cellular steady state levels of Type I procollagen mRNAs in both chick skin and lung fibroblasts (36). However, increases of procollagen mRNAs were observed in the polysomal fraction (Figure 3). Both nuclear and post-polysomal cytoplasmic Type I procollagen mRNAs were significantly decreased after bleomycin treatment. Accordingly, bleomycin treatment of chick skin and lung fibroblasts resulted in a redistribution of Type I procollagen mRNAs within the nuclear, post-polysomal cytoplasmic and polysomal subcellular fractions.

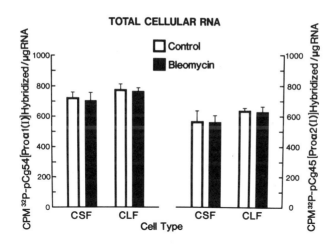

Figure 2: Lack of effect of bleomycin on steady state total cellular levels of Type 1 procollagen mRNAs. Chick skin and chick lung fibroblasts were grown to late log phase and treated with bleomycin. After 48 hr the cells were collected and total cellular RNA was isolated. The steady state levels of Type I procollagen mRNAs were determined by dot blot hybridization using recombinant cDNA probes. The values represent the mean ± S.E. of 3-6 separate experiments.

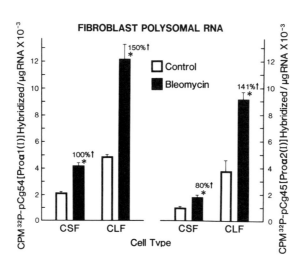

<u>Figure 3</u>:   Bleomycin-induced polysomal partitioning of
Type I procollagen mRNAs.   Chick lung and chick skin
fibroblasts were grown to late log phase and treated for
48 hr with bleomycin. The cells were harvested, polysomes were isolated and polysomal RNA was extracted.   The
concentrations of Type I procollagen mRNAs were determined by dot blot hybridization. The values represent the
mean ± S.E. of 3-6 separate experiments.

There are precedents in the literature for a polysomal partitioning effect similar to that caused by
bleomycin. A partitioning of poly(A)RNAs into the
polysomes of BALB/c 3T3 cells occurs after serum stimulation (37, 38). Furthermore, the thyrotropin-stimulated

synthesis of thyroglobulin in ox and dog thyroid slices is accompanied by an increase in thyroglobulin synthesizing polysomes which is mediated by a shift of inactive thyroglobulin mRNA into membrane bound polysomes (39). These studies indicate that increased translation of a specific mRNA is not necessarily accompanied by an increase in transcription but may be dependent on the activation of existing cellular mRNAs under the control of a specific translational factor(s). Future studies of this polysomal partitioning phenomenon may elucidate a unique mechanism of regulation of procollagen synthesis at the translational level and may provide a molecular basis for the initiation and progression of fibrotic lung disease.

Glucocorticoids have been shown to selectively decrease collagen synthesis in tissues and in cells (for review see 40). Dexamethasone treatment of primary chick skin fibroblasts decreased the steady state levels of Type I procollagen mRNAs (41). This glucocorticoid-mediated decrease in cellular levels of Type I procollagen mRNAs was associated with a temporal decrease of these mRNAs in the nucleus, cytoplasm and polysomes. Type I procollagen hnRNAs were also decreased in dexamethasone-treated chick skin fibroblasts. These dexamethasone-induced decreases of Type I procollagen mRNAs result from a decrease of Type I procollagen gene expression.

As seen in Figure 4 simultaneous treatment of chick skin and lung fibroblasts with bleomycin and dexamethasone prevented the bleomycin-induced increase of procollagen synthesis. In addition, this corticosteroid also prevented the polysomal partitioning of Type I procollagen mRNAs. This finding at least in part may explain the ability of glucocorticoids to inhibit the bleomycin-induced increase of proteinaceous hydroxyproline and collagen synthesis in lung in vivo.

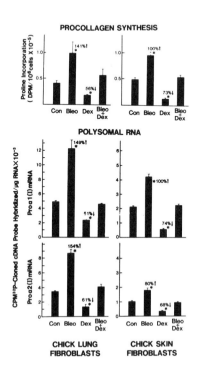

<u>Figure 4</u>: Dexamethasone inhibition of the bleomycin-induced increase of procollagen synthesis and Type I procollagen mRNA polysomal partitioning. Chick lung and chick skin fibroblasts were grown to late log phase and treated with bleomycin, dexamethasone or bleomycin plus dexamethasone. Some cells were labeled with [³H] proline and collagen and noncollagen protein synthesis was determined by the collagenase assay. Other cells were homogenized and polysomes were isolated. Polysomal RNA was extracted and the concentration of Type I procollagen mRNAs were determined by the dot blot assay. Incorporation data represents the mean ± S.E of 3-5 cultures. Type I procollagen mRNA data represent the mean ± S.E. of 3-6 experiments. (Reprinted with permission from ref. 40).

The direct effect of bleomycin on cultured fibro-blasts, resulting in the polysomal partitioning of Type I procollagen mRNAs constitutes one potential mechanism of bleomycin-induced pulmonary fibrosis. Other nonexclusive potential mechanisms of pulmonary fibrosis are genetic predisposition or the effect of bleomycin-induced pulmonary fibrosis on various cell types in the lung to produce factors which regulate fibroblast growth and fibroblast function.

REFERENCES:

1. Hussar, D.A. Am. J. Pharm. 146: 37-58, 1974.
2. Muller, W.E.G., Yamazaki, Z., Breter, H.J. and Zahn, R.K. Eur. J. Biochem. 31: 518-525, 1972.
3. Sausville, E.A., Peisach, J. and Horwitz, S.B. Biochemistry 17: 2740-2746, 1978.
4. Sausville, E.A., Stein, R.W., Peisach, J. and Horwitz, S.B. Biochemistry 17: 2746-2754, 1978.
5. Suzuki, H., Nagai, K., Yamaki, H., Tanaka, N. and Umezawa, H. J. Antibiot. 21: 379-386, 1968.
6. Muller, W.E.G., Totsuka, A., Nusser, I., Zahn, R.K. and Umezawa, H. Biochem. Pharmacol. 24: 911-915, 1975.
7. Takeshita, M., Horwitz, S.B. and Grollman, A.P. Virology 60: 455-465, 1974.
8. Kuo, M.T. and Haidle, C.W. Biochem. Biophys. Acta 335: 109-114, 1974.
9. Haidle, C.W. and Lloyd, R.S. In: Bleomycin: Current Status and New Development Eds. S. K. Carter, S. T. Crooke and H. Umezawa), Academic Press, New York, N. Y., 1978, p. 21.
10. Kuo, M.T. Cancer Res. 41: 2439-2443, 1981.
11. Adamson, I.Y.R. Environ. Health Perspect. 16: 119-126, 1976.
12. Bedrossian, C.W.M., Greenberg, S.D., Yawn, D.H. and O'Neal, R.M. Arch. Pathol. and Lab. Med. 101: 248-254, 1977.
13. Snider, G.L., Hayes, J.A. and Korthy, A.L. Am. Rev. Resp. Dis. 117: 1099-1108, 1978.
14. Giri, S.N., Schwartz, L.W., Hollinger, M.A., Freywald, M.E., Schiedt, M.J. and Zuckerman, J.E. Exptl. and Mol. Pathol. 33: 1-14, 1980.
15. Lazo, J.S. and Humphreys, C.J. Proc. Natl. Acad. Sci. 80: 3064-3068, 1983.
16. McCullough, B., Collins, J.F., Johanson W.G. and Grover, F.L. J. Clin. Invest. 61: 79-88, 1978.
17. Sikic, B.I., Young, D.M., Mimmaugh, E.G. and Gram, T.E. Cancer Res. 38: 787-792, 1978.
18. Starcher, B.C., Kuhn, C. and Overton, J.E. Amer. Rev. Resp. Dis. 117: 299-305, 1978.
19. Goldstein, R.H., Lucey, E.C., Franzblau, C. and Snider, G.L. Amer. Rev. Resp. Dis. 120: 67-73, 1979.
20. Sterling, K.M., DiPetrillo, T., Cutroneo, K.R. and Prestayko, A. Cancer Res. 42: 405-408, 1982.
21. Zapol, W.M., Trelstad, R.L., Coffey, J.W., Tsai, I. and Salvador, R.A. Am. Rev. Resp. Dis. 119: 547-554, 1979.

22. Clark, J.G., Overton, J.E., Marino, B.A., Uitto, J. and Starcher, B.C. J. Lab. Clin. Med. 96: 943-953, 1980.
23. Phan, S.H., Thrall, R.S. and Ward, P.A. Am. Rev. Resp. Dis. 121: 501-506, 1980.
24. Zuckerman, J.E., Hollinger, M.A. and Giri, S.N. J. Pharmacol. Exptl. Therapeu. 213: 425-431 (1980).
25. Laurent, G. and McAnulty, R.J. Am. Rev. Respir. Dis. 128: 82-88, 1983.
26. Cantor, J. O., Cerreta, J.M., Osman, M., Mott, S.H., Mandl, I. and Turino, G.M. Proc. Soc. Exptl. Biol. and Med. 174: 172-181, 1983.
27. Counts, D.F., Evans, J.N., DiPetrillo, T.A., Sterling, K.M. and Kelley, J. J. Pharmacol. and Exptl. Therapeu. 219: 675-678, 1981.
28. Sterling, K.M., DiPetrillo, T.A., Kotch J.P. and Cutroneo, K.R. Cancer Res. 42: 3502-3506, 1982.
29. Clark, J.G., Starcher, B.C. and Uitto, J. Biochem. Biophys. Acta 631: 359-370, 1980.
30. Clark, J.G., Kostal, K.M. and Marino, B.A. J. Clin. Invest. 72: 2082-2091, 1983.
31. Bitterman, P.B., Adelberg, S. and Crystal, R.G. J. Clin. Invest. 72: 1801-1813, 1983.
32. Kovacs, E.J. and Kelley, J. J. Leuk. Biol. 37: 1-14, 1985.
33. Kovacs E.J. and Kelley, J. Am. Rev. Respir. Dis. 133: 68-72, 1986.
34. Kovacs, E.J. and Kelley, J. Am. J. Pathol. 121: 261-268, 1985.
35. Clark, J.G., Kostal, K.M. and Marino, B.A. J. Biol. Chem. 257: 8098-8105, 1982.
36. Sterling, K.M., Harris, M.J., Mitchell, J.J. and Cutroneo, K.R. J. Biol. Chem. 258: 14438-14444, 1983.
37. Bandman, E. and Gurney, T. Jr. Exptl. Cell Res. 90: 159-168, 1975.
38. Rudland, P.S., Weil, S. and Hunter, A.R. J. Mol. Biol. 96: 745-766, 1975.
39. Davies, E., Dumont, J.E. and Vassart, G. Biochem. J. 172: 227-231, 1978.
40. Cutroneo, K.R., Sterling, K.M. and Shull, S. In: Biology of Extracellular Matrix (Ed. R. P. Mecham), Academic Press, New York, N.Y., 1986, pp. 119-176.
41. Cockayne, D., Sterling, K.M. Jr., Shull, S., Mintz, K.P., Illeyne S. and Cutroneo, K.R. Biochem. 25: 3202-3209, 1986.

SECTION III

PLATINUM INDUCED NEPHROTOXICITY

Chaired by M.P. Hacker

Overview
M.P. Hacker

Since Rosenberg's initial observation in the 1960's that diamminedichloroplatinum (II) (DDP) was cytotoxic to bacterial and mammalian cells, DDP has become one of the most widely used anticancer drugs. As with all cancer chemotherapeutic agents, DDP causes significant toxicity to the patient, including myelosuppression, nausea, vomiting, nephrotoxicity, ototoxicity, peripheral neuropathy, tetany and allergic reactions. The objective of this session was to focus on the nephrotoxicity of DDP and to discuss possible mechanisms and approaches to diminishing this dose limiting, untoward effect of DDP.

While a number of possible mechanisms such as membrane effects, enzyme inhibition, altered cellular metabolism or electrolyte imbalance have been proposed, none has been adequate to totally explain the nephrotoxicity of DDP. Recent results emanating from several laboratories suggest that perhaps platinum-DNA interactions may be playing a role in DDP induced kidney damage. Using an enzyme linked immunosorbent assay (ELISA), a relatively new technique to determine the extent of intrastrand crosslinks, Dr. Litterst reported that the kidney accumulates more DNA adducts then either gonadal tissue or tumor. He further found that adducts which were formed remained stable for at least fourteen days. A number of factors including diet, gender, castration and dose had significant effects on total platinum and/or DNA adduct formation.

Taking a different approach, Dr. Safirstein reported on the effects of biochemical and physiological DDP on the kidney function. Physiological effects can be divided into three distinct phases that persist for up to four weeks following a single DDP injection. A component seen throughout the disease process is polyuria. The mechanism of this uniform response to DDP administration remains an active area of research. DDP also inhibits renal energy metabolism. However, data presented by Dr. Safirstein suggest that this effect may not be important in the early pathogenesis of kidney damage. Finally, in a series of experiments, Safirstein demonstrated that DDP causes increased DNA turnover and oncogene expression in renal tissue. These effects need further study to determine their role in DDP induced kidney damage.

The use of pharmacological interventions to diminish DDP renal damage has been the focus of research in a number of laboratories. In his presentation, Dr. Borch reviewed the current status of three potentially important chemoprotectors. Thiosulfate, diethyldithiocarbamate (DDTC), and WR2721 have all proven effective in preclinical studies and are now in various stages of clinical evaluation. Using a renal epithelial cell line, Borch and his co-workers have begun to investigate the mechanistic basis of DDP nephrotoxicity and DDTC protection. These studies suggest that of the three chemoprotectants only DDTC is truly capable of rescuing renal tissue. Which of these protectants will ultimately provide the greatest clinical utility is unknown.

Hydration and osmotic diuresis have decreased nephrotoxicity when low levels of DDP are used. However, escalation beyond 130-140 mg/m^2 have not been routinely possible. Using hypertonic saline at the time of DDP administration and maintaining vigorous chloruresis, Ozols and his colleagues have been able to administer 200 mg/m^2 total dose DDP without concomitant nephrotoxicity. Encouraging results are being obtained in heavily pretreated ovarian cancer patients and high risk testicular cancer patients. Using the ELISA assay for intrastrand crosslinks, their group has been able to correlate clinical response and possibly toxicity with adduct formation in WBC and target tissue, respectively. In spite of high dose DDP no significant renal toxicity has been observed. Rather, the dose limiting toxicity appears now to be peripheral neuropathy. The mechanism of neurotoxicity is unknown but may be related to Schwann cell loss.

A number of posters concerning DDP toxicity were presented. A series of posters reported the effects on renal function in which the primary acute change appears to be in the proximal tubule with subsequent decrease in glomerular filtration rate. A major focus of the poster presentations was the use of chemoprotectants. Such nucleophiles as glutathione, DDTC, thiosulfate and disulfiram were studied. An exciting clinical observation was the fact that reduced glutathione prevented not only nephrotoxicity but neurotoxicity, as well. This potentially important observation needs further investigation.

Other toxic effects of DDP including pulmonary damage, ototoxicity and vestibular toxicity were also presented. DDP appears to enhance the lung damaging effects of bleomycin possibly by altering kidney function. Ototoxicity may be modulated by melanin concentration and may be preventable with a new phosphonic acid antibiotic, fosfomycin. A new method for testing vestibular toxicity was presented and is currently being evaluated for clinical application. The localization of platinum in the kidney was studied in rats administered DDP, iproplatin or paraplatin. DDP was retained in the pars recta for a more prolonged time than either of the other two drugs. Chronic nephrotoxicity following DDP administration in germ cell patients was evidenced by prolonged hypomagnesemia. Also, increased cumulative DDP dose resulted in increased chronic serum hypomagnesemia.

Factors Influencing the Formation and Persistence of Platinum-DNA Adducts in Tissues of Rats Treated with Cisplatin
C.L. Litterst, M.C. Poirier, E. Reed

INTRODUCTION

The importance of cisplatin as a cancer chemotherapeutic agent has become increasingly obvious during the past 10-15 years. Studies of the mechanism of action of this compound predate clinical studies and established very early that the antitumor effect of cisPt was due to its ability to inhibit DNA synthesis. Further studies established the probability that DNA inhibition was caused by formation of a bidentate link between the de-chlorinated cisPt molecule and nucleophilic sites on the DNA strand, likely to be either N^7 or O^6 of the guanine base. Recent studies by several groups (1-3) have shown that the platinum-DNA linkage is predominantly between two guanine bases (G-G) and between adenine and guanine (A-G) on the same DNA strand (intrastrand cross link) and these intrastrand links correlate closely with antitumor efficacy and DNA inhibition.

The potential involvement of the Pt-DNA complex in the organ-specific toxicity of cisPt has been largely overlooked, however, as investigators focused on cisPt interactions with sulfhydryl compounds (4,5) or enzymes (6,7) as possible molecular mechanisms to explain the compromised renal function and severe gastrointestinal toxicity that characterizes cisPt toxicity in both animals and humans.

The possibility that cisPt organ-specific toxicity might involve DNA interaction initially occurred to us after it became apparent that the toxic effects of cisPt on the kidney did not occur immediately upon drug injection. Even at cisPt doses of 30 mg/kg--4-5 times the acute median lethal dose-only occasional deaths occur prior to day 3 and none occur prior to day 2. Furthermore, when in vivo clearance studies of either inulin or cisPt were conducted, studies were either negative or equivocal until 36-48 hr after cisPt dosing, at which time clearance values dropped dramatically. These latter results were reported independently by Saferstein and colleagues using micropuncture techniques to study renal function (8). The common denominator of these toxicity studies and nucleic acid involvement is the fact that in a some mammalian cells, a complete cell cycle requires around 24 hours (9), suggesting that whatever the mechanisms of cisPt toxicity it somehow may involve 1 or 2 cycles of cell replication to become manifest as an observable change in renal cell homeostasis. This is similar to the single cycle of cell replication required to fix the initiating event in chemical carcinogenesis(10).

Until recently our ability to study Pt-DNA interaction at any quantitatively significant level was severely limited by the lack of sensitivity of traditional analytical methods. The limit of sensitivity of conventional atomic absorption spectroscopy (AAS), for example, is on the order of 1 ng of platinum, which means that relatively high levels of platination of the DNA molecule are required in order for us to be able to detect a Pt-DNA interaction. Recently antibodies have been produced that are specific for the platinum G-G and A-G intrastrand crosslink (1,2). This innovation has provided platinum sensitivity that is on the order of femtomoles of Pt per ug of DNA. This low level detection of platinum bound to DNA now provides the analytical means of permitting us to investigate whether or not the Pt-DNA interaction may, in fact, be involved with producing the renal toxicity and what the exact role of the adduct is. Prior to actual mechanism of action studies our approach has been to characterize the Pt-DNA adducts as they occur in animals following cisplatin administration. This paper will report results of these studies on the relation between Pt-DNA adducts and normal parameters of toxicity and pharmacokinetics.

METHODS

General

Adult male and female Sprague Dawley rats were injected either ip or iv with cisPt prepared in 0.9% NaCl. Except for several early experiments animals were routinely fasted overnight prior to drug injection. Rats routinely were killed by ether overdose 4 hr after drug treatment, except in experiments to determine stability of the adducts, in which case animals were killed 4 hr, 1,2,3 weeks following dosing. Blood was drawn from the vena cava and tissues were removed and immediately frozen on dry ice. Samples were stored at -70^0 until analysis. Tissues were homogenized (1:3) in 0.25% triton X-100 and the homogenate or plasma analyzed for total platinum content by conventional AAS. Nonprotein sulfhydryl (NPS) content of tissue was determined by homogenizing ice cold tissue samples in 10 volumes of 5% trichloroacetic acid. The supernatant after centrifugation was analyzed for NPS by the method of Ellman (11). Early studies compared the results of NPS determination with those when oxidized and reduced glutathione were determined. No differences in results were found (data not presented) so NPS values were routinely determined. Urea nitrogen values in plasma (BUN) were assayed using a reagent kit (Sigma Chem. Co., St. Louis, MO)

In studies utilizing castrated animals, surgical removal of testes through an incision in the scrotum or removal of the ovaries through a dorsal abdominal wall incision was followed by 2 weeks of recovery prior to drug administration. In these experiments, weights of seminal vesicles and uteri, as well as plasma concentrations of testosterone, progesterone, and estrogen were determined to establish efficacy of the castration.

Renal clearance of platinum during a steady state infusion of cisplatin was conducted as described previously (12). Briefly, rats were anesthetized and cannulae inserted into the femoral vein and artery, and the ureter of one kidney. After an intravenous loading dose, a constant rate infusion was established. Fifteen minute urine collections were made with an arterial blood sample taken at the midpoint of the urine collection period.

Adduct Determination.

The technique for determining the presence of Pt-DNA intrastrand cross-links is a competitive ELISA previously published in detail (1). In brief non-platinated or variously platinated (0-4.3%) calf thymus DNA is coated on microtiter plate wells. Either sample DNA or platinated calf thymus DNA is then incubated with excess antibody specific for the Pt-DNA adduct, and the competition is allowed to come to equilibrium during a 90 minute incubation at 37⁰. Aliquots of this antigen-antibody mixture then were placed into microtiter plate wells and incubated for an additional 90 min. Excess antibody then binds to the DNA coated on the plate wells. Everything not bound to the microtiter well is removed by washing with buffer, and the amount of antibody that is bound to the well is determined by addition to the microtiter plate of an alkaline phosphatase conjugate that interacts with the bound antibody. After washing, p-nitrophenyl phosphate is added and the hydrolysis to p-nitrophenol (PNP) measured spectrophotometrically. The PNP quantity is in direct proportion to the quantity of antibody present in the microtiter plate well. The assay is standardized against an in vitro-modified cisplatin-DNA, the platinum content of which is determined by AAS. The antibody, however, does not recognize all of the platinum bound to DNA. Preliminary studies suggest that the tertiary structure of the in vivo modified DNA is different from that of the highly modified immunogen. Preliminary experiments have demonstrated about a 1000-fold higher platinum-DNA concentration measurable by AAS as compared to the DNA adducts measurable by the ELISA in the same biological samples. * Therefore, the ELISA values reported in this paper as attomoles/ ug DNA are an underestimation of the total intrastrand adduct quantities. Studies are underway to better define the nature of that portion of the adduct that the antibody recognizes. A more quantitative radio-immunoassay is being developed that will be used to confirm the in vivo results presented here.

RESULTS

At the beginning of these experiments, the data showed large inter-and intra-experiment variability. Thus values from week to

*Personal communication (A.M. Fichtinger-Schepmah).

week and from animal to animal varied widely, often over a range of 5x or more. In an attempt to identify the primary cause for this variability we ran an experiment wherein some animals were fasted overnight and others were allowed free access to food. The primary finding from this experiment (Table 1) was that variability was not reduced by fasting, as seen by the large standard deviations

Table 1. Influence of fasting on Pt-DNA adduct levels in rats 4 hour after iv injection of cisplatin (8 mg/kg)

	FED	FASTED
Kidney adducts (attmol/ug DNA)	520 + 60	900 + 140
Kidney total platinum (ug/g)	45 + 3	51 + 5
Urinary excretion (% Dose)	19 + 3	24 + 3

in adduct levels in fasted animals. In fact, variability appeared to be greater in the fasted group than in the fed group. In addition, there were no differences in renal or plasma total platinum levels nor, surprisingly, in renal or plasma NPS levels. However it can be seen that renal adduct levels were twice as great in fasted animals as in fed animals. Although there is a large amount of variability within the groups, similar large variability was less apparent with both urinary platinum excretion or renal total platinum levels.

Using fasted animals because of the higher adduct levels that are formed we then investigated the effect of route of administration on adduct formation. This time we extended our observations to include adduct levels in testes as well as those in kidney and compared iv with ip drug administration. No significant differences were found between the two routes of administration (data not shown). This result is not particularly surprising in light of the rapid uptake of drugs from the peritoneal cavity and the large body of data showing similar distribution of drugs administered by these two

routes. It is of interest to note that testicular adduct levels
(21-26 attmol/ug DNA) were only about 1/3 as great as renal adduct
levels (83-86 attmol/ug DNA).

We then were interested in the amount of adduct that accumulated
in solid tumors relative to normal tissues. Female rats carrying a
3-5 g solid Walker 256 carcinosarcoma tumor subcutaneously in the
flank were injected with a very high dose of cisPt (30 mg/kg) and
adduct levels compared between tumor and kidney. Tumor adduct levels
(458 ± 45 attmol/ug DNA) were about 1/3 of those in kidney (1220 ± 170
attmol/ug DNA), a ratio similar to that seen between testes and
kidney.

Table 2. Pt-DNA adduct levels in tissues of male and female rats 4
hours after intraperitoneal injection of cisplatin.

	Dose (mg/kg)	Renal Pt (ug/g)	Adducts (attmol/ug DNA)	
			Kidney	Gonad
Female	10	25 ± 5	1522 ± 210	ND
	30	66 ± 9	3900 ± 470	80 ± 30
Male	10	30 ± 3	2550 ± 560	140 ± 30
	30	79 ± 5	6500 ± 410	160 ± 50

ND = None Detected (< 25 attmol/ug DNA)

A direct comparison was then conducted using male and female
rats injected ip with aliquots from the same drug solution at two
different doses of cisPt. Renal total platinum levels in this experiment were the same in both sexes (Table 2). However it can be observed that renal adduct levels were significantly greater in males than
in females by nearly 70%. Gonadal levels of adducts were substant-

ially less than renal adduct levels and were greater in males than in females. Although a dose-response is suggested for renal adduct formation, no similar relation is observed for testes adduct formation.

In order to investigate the effect of sex hormones on adduct formation, we repeated the above study two weeks after surgical castration of rats. In males, castration made no difference in levels of adducts, even though decreases in serum testosterone levels and in seminal vesicle weights indicated that castration had been complete (Table 3). In females, however, castration resulted in nearly a 50% increase in adduct formation in kidney. Because of the complexity of female hormone production, serum hormone levels and uterine weights were not reduced completely to zero. A more complete time course after castration might have revealed different results if the study had been done 4-6 weeks after ovariectomy. The reason for the increase in adduct formation when total platinum renal levels were not elevated may be related to observed serum progesterone levels and is the focus of continuing work in our laboratories.

Table 3. Effect of castration on kidney levels of Pt-DNA adducts 4 hours after 20 mg/kg cisplatin ip.

	FEMALES				
	Adducts (amol/ug)	Total Pt (ug/g)	Progest. (ng/ml)	Estrogens (pg/ml)	Uterus (mg)
Sham	280 + 20	23 + 3	28 + 4	80 + 9	290 + 10
Castrated	400 + 50	27 + 4	10 + 1	65 + 2	110 + 5

	MALES			
	Adducts (amol/ug)	Total Pt (ug/g)	Testost. (ng/ml)	Semin. Vesic. (mg)
Sham	1450 + 260	35 + 1	8 + 1	750 + 30
Castrated	1270 + 200	29 + 4	0.1	60 + 4

We then conducted a comprehensive dose response study that covered the dose range from 5-30 mg/kg. As shown in Figure 1, total platinum levels in both kidney and gonad from males and females showed the expected increase in concentration with increasing dose. Renal adducts increased continually beginning at 10 mg/kg, with a relatively sharper increase at 30 mg/kg than expected from mere extrapolation from the 20 mg/kg dose. Gonadal adduct levels were relatively low, with no adducts detectable in ovaries below 30 mg/kg. Testicular Pt-DNA adducts were routinely higher than those in ovary, but did not demonstrate a detectable increase with dose until 30 mg/kg.

The retention of Pt-DNA adducts then was the focus of our attention. After a single bolus injection, the time course of disappearance of adducts is shown in Figure 2. In all cases except ovary, there was an apparent increase in adduct concentration between the time of injection (4 hr) and our analysis point two days later. After that time, renal and gonadal adduct levels decreased, with 29-33% of maximal levels still remaining in male tissues two weeks after injection. A similar time course of adduct retention was im-

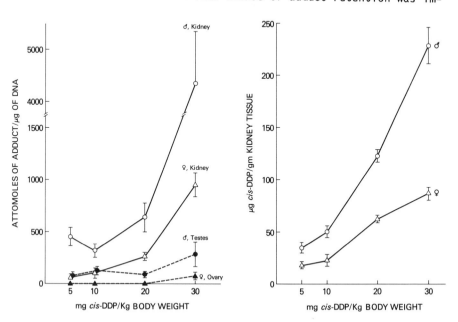

Figure 1. Accumulation of total platinum (right) and Pt-DNA adducts (left) with increasing dose [14].

possible to conduct in female rats due to an increased sensitivity of the female to the lethal effects of cisPt. Thus by day 11 all of the female rats injected with a second 5 mg/kg dose of cisPt had died, whereas only 33% of the male rats similarly injected had died, thus leaving several males available for study on day 14. In the females at day 7, however, 23% of the renal adducts remained while greater than half of the adducts present in ovary were still present.

As an aside, we briefly investigated the sex difference in sensitivity to cisPt. We had observed that survival of female Sprague Dawley rats always was less than survival of male Sprague Dawleys

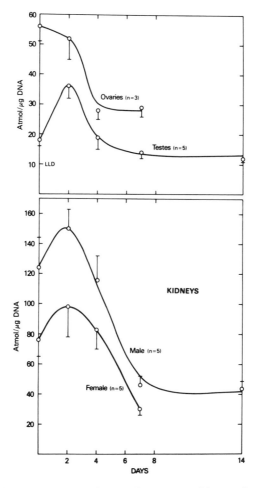

Figure 2.   Stability of Pt-DNA adducts in rat
             kidney (lower) and gonads (upper).

injected with the same dose of cisplatin. In addition, BUN elevations routinely occurred earlier and were greater with females than with males, even though kidney total platinum concentrations were similar for both sexes (data not presented). This latter fact suggests that differences in end-organ sensitivity might be the reason for the difference in sensitivity, or that a target organ other than kidney may be involved with causing death. However, when the retention of total platinum following a single 8 mg/kg dose was studied in both sexes, there was a suggestion of higher plasma total Pt concentration in females throughout the 7 days of the study. When data from the dose response experiment then was carefully examined it was obvious that,indeed, plasma concentrations of platinum were consistently greater in females than was observed for the same dose in males. We therefore conducted a brief study to examine the in vivo renal clearance of platinum following cisPt administration. In females renal clearance of Pt was 0.39 ± 0.14 ml/min (n=6) and in two males the value was 1.1 ± 0.2 ml/min. This value for males agreed well with previously published clearance values in male rats (12) and so no additional animals were studied. It therefore appears as if cisPt is cleared by the female kidney at about half or less of the rate of clearance by the male kidney. This difference might expose renal tubules to a higher concentration of Pt for a longer time, which might account for the increased sensitivity of females.

Table 4. Accumulation of Pt-DNA adducts in kidneys of male rats 4 hour after each of 2 weekly 5 mg/kg injections of cisplatin

	Kidney		Plasma
	Adducts (attmol/ug)	Total Pt (ug/g)	Total Pt (ug/ml)
Week 1	665 ± 82	8.3 ± 0.3	1.3 ± 0.1
2	451 ± 67	10.9 ± 1.0	1.4 ± 0.2

Representative results of several experiments designed to study the accumulation of adducts following multiple weekly injections of cisplatin are shown in Table 4. Renal concentrations of total platinum increased as would be expected for a highly retained molecule like platinum. However, Pt-DNA adducts levels are lower 4 hr after the second injection than they were 4 hr after the first injection. Because separate groups of rats were injected and sacrificed at each time it could be argued that the lower adduct levels found after the first injection were due to an injection error. However, in at least 3 separate replicates of this experiment, similar results have been obtained. The reason for this apparent decreased concentration of adducts is unknown. It may be that the adducts measured 4 hr after drug injection have not yet become fully fixed in the DNA molecule and thus are not representative of true adducts. Also, it may be that the second dose of cisplatin stimulates extensive DNA repair, such that a portion of adducts remaining from the first injection also are removed. Another possibility is that cells with the highest adduct levels die first and are sloughed into the tubular lumen and lost in the urine.

In all studies conducted in this series of experiments and reported here, BUN and NPS were routinely determined. BUN showed the expected increase with time after treatment and dose in the dose response and retention/ accumulation studies. However, differences were observed between male and female rats, as discussed above. NPS, which we hoped might show a correlation with adduct levels and/or toxicity were uniformly unchanged in most of the work we did and thus provided no help in suggesting a mechanism of action or potential involvement with adduct formation or toxicity.

DISCUSSION

It is apparent from these results that adducts between cisplatin and DNA form in both tumor tissue and nontumor normal tissues and are stable for at least 14 days and probably much longer. Kidney accumulates greater numbers of adducts than testes or ovaries and tumor contains about the same adduct levels as were observed in gonads.

For the same dose of cisplatin there is a higher concentration of adducts in male kidney than in female kidney and the male gonad also has higher levels than does the female gonad. Total kidney platinum concentration however are not significantly different between the two sexes. The reason for this gender-related difference in adduct formation relative to total amount of platinum is unknown and is in contrast to the apparent greater sensitivity of the female Sprague Dawley rat to the lethal effect of cisplatin. Castration increased the formation of adducts in the female but not to levels found in the males, while the presence of testosterone has no significant impact on adduct levels in male kidney. Thus the role of hormone levels is still uncertain.

When we investigated the ability of kidney and gonads to accumulate Pt-DNA adducts following repeated low doses of cisPt, we found a surprise. Rather than having progressively greater quantities of adducts in tissues, there appeared to be a smaller concentration of adducts after the second injection than was present after the first injection. Because of the total platinum retention curves, we expected that one week after injection there should be at least as many adducts as were present initially. The results of these studies with multiple injections suggest that there may be a control mechanism which regulates the amount of platinum present in kidney at any one time, or may regulate the formation of adducts. This would then appear inconsistent with the dose response study, which showed an increase in both adducts and total platinum with increasing dose. Perhaps there is a mechanism which controls adducts formation when "old" adducts are still present, but which does not operate--or not as efficiently--when a large amount of platinum is presented to the tissues at one time. Similar studies have beeen conducted in guinea pigs with sequential treatment separated by 1,2,or 3 days rather than weekly (13). Results of the guinea pig study showed that total platinum levels in kidney were increased when injections were separated by one day but there was no significant increase in total platinum levels when injections were separated by 2 days.

Our work has demonstrated that cisplatin forms stable adducts with DNA in normal tissues of animals. The relationship, if any, between these adducts and the organ-specific toxicity of this drug is still unknown, however, and a topic for continued investigation.

REFERENCES
1. Poirier MC, SJ Lippard, LA Zwelling, HM Ushay, D Kerrigan, CC Thill, SM Santela, D Grunberger, SH Yuspa (1982), Proc. Nat. Acad. Sci.79:6443-47.
2. Plooy, ACM, AMJ Fichtinger-Shepman, HH Schutte, M van Dijk, PHM Lohman (1985), Carcinogenesis 6:561-566.
3. Lippard, SJ, HM Ushay, CM Merkel, MC Poirier (1983) Biochem. 22: 5165-68.
4. Litterst, CL, In: Biochemical Mechanisms of Platinum Antitumour Drugs (DCH McBrien & TF Slater, eds) IRL Press, Oxford, 1986, pp pp 227-254.
5. Levi, J, C Jacobs, S Kalman, M McTigue, M Winer (1980), J. Pharmacol. exptl. Therapeut. 213:545-550.
6. Uozumi, J & CL Litterst, (1985) Cancer Chemother Pharmacol 15:93-6.
7. Aull, JL, RL Allen, AR Bapat, HH Daron, ME Friedman, JF Wilson (1979) Biochem Biophys Acta 571:352-358.
8. Saferstein, R, P Miller, S Dikman, N Lyman & C Shapiro (1981), Am J Physiol 41:F175-179.
9. Guiguet, M, J-J Kupiec, A-J Valleran, In: Cell Cycle Clocks (LN Edmunds, ed) M. Dekker, NY 1984, pp 97-111.
10. Farber, E & DSR Sarma (1987) Lab. Invest. 56:4-22.
11. Ellman, GL (1959) Arch Biochem Biophys 82:70-77.
12. Osman, N & CL Litterst (1983), Cancer Lett 19:107-111.
13. Litterst, CL & VG Schweitzer (1984) Cancer Chemother Pharmacol 12: 12:46-49.
14. Reed, E, CL Litterst, C Thill, S Yuspa, & M Poirier (1987) Cancer Res 47:718-722.

Cisplatin Nephrotoxicity: New Insights Into Mechanism
R. Safirstein, A.Z. Zelent, and R. Gordon

Cis-dichlorodiammine platinum (II), or cisplatin, has emerged as a principal chemotherapeutic agent in the treatment of otherwise resistant solid tumors and is currently among the most widely used agents in the chemotherapy of cancer. The chief limit to its greater efficacy, however, is its nephrotoxicity, which has made it necessary both to lower its dosage and actively hydrate patients to reduce it. These techniques have proven to be only partially successful as renal failure occurs even at such low doses and especially after its repeated administration (1,2). Use of other means to protect the kidney (3-5) are only partially successful and of uncertain clinical application. It may not be possible to alter or prevent the renal toxicity of cisplatin, however, until a more basic understanding of that toxicity is obtained. This paper summarizes what is known about the biochemical and physiologic aspects of cisplatin nephrotoxicity and gives the results of some recent experiments into its possible mechanism.

A. Renal uptake, excretion, and metabolism of cisplatin

The kidney is the principal excretory organ of cisplatin. In the rat, 50% of injected cisplatin is excreted in the urine 24 hours after its administration (6) and most of excreted platinum appears in the urine within the first hour (7). Unbound cisplatin is freely filtered at the glomerulus (8) and may be secreted onto the urine as well (9, 10). There does not seem to be a significant reabsorptive flux of cisplatin, as microinjected cisplatin is almost completely recovered in the urine (11).

The renal concentration of platinum is several fold above plasma levels and above that in other organs (6). Almost all of the platinum in the kidney is contained within the cortex and can be found in all subcellular organelles as well as the cytosole (7). The process by which the kidney accumulates cisplatin is dependent upon normal oxygen utilization (8) and is partially inhibitable by drugs that compete for the transport of organic bases in a dose dependent manner. Drugs that compete for the organic anion transport system, such as PAH and pyrazinoic acid, do not inhibit uptake. Taken together, these observations suggest that the renal uptake of cisplatin involves some specific interaction of the drug with the kidney, perhaps involving transport or binding to components of the base transport system. The data also suggest that platinum gains access to the renal cell from the peritubular, rather than the urinary, aspect of the cell.

Cisplatin is excreted largely unchanged in the urine (8). Upon entry into the renal cell, however, cisplatin undergoes biotransformation. In addition to binding to cell macromolecules, a large portion (30-50%) of the total cell platinum is in a form whose molecular weight is below 500 daltons and whose chromatographic behavior is different from cisplatin. Another characteristic of this platinum metabolite is the loss of its biologic activity as a mutagen. Whereas excreted platinum is mutagenic (12), cell platinum is not. As the mutagenic activity of platinum coordination complexes is correlated with their cellular toxicity (13), the loss of mutagenicity by renal cell platinum suggests a loss of toxicity. Confirmation of this will require isolation and identification of this compound.

B. Physiologic aspects of cisplatin-induced nephrotoxicity

After a single 5 mg/kg body weight (BW) dose to rat, cisplatin produces renal failure in three distinct phases (14): 1) an induction phase (48 hours), when polyuria occurs without a fall in GFR; 2) a maintenance phase (72h-2weeks), when azotemia and polyuria coexist; 3) and a partial recovery phase (up to four weeks), when blood urea nitrogen (BUN) returns to normal but polyuria and reduced glomerular filtration persists.

Reduced renal plasma flow and elevated renal vascular resistance, as well as a reduced glomerular ultrafiltration coefficient (K_f), may all participate in the fall of GFR (15). Rapid infusion of isoncotic albumin reverses some of these changes only partially indicating persistent high renovascular resistance. Identification of the mediator of these intrarenal vascular effects is still an active area of research but studies to date have ruled out a prominent role for angiotensin or adenosine in the low GFR after cisplatin treatment (11).

Polyuria uniformly accompanies cisplatin administration and occurs in two distinct stages. Urine osmolality initially falls over the first 24-48 hours after cisplatin is given, but GFR in this stage is normal. This early polyuria usually ameliorates spontaneously and responds to large doses of vasopressin (16). A second stage, characterized by increased volume and reduced osmolality, occurs between 72 and 96 h and persists for at least one month after exposure to cisplatin. This later stage is accompanied by reduced GFR and does not respond to vasopressin. Neither elevated rates of fluid and solute flows from superficial nephrons, nor an altered ability to generate a normal transepithelial solute gradient at the thick ascending limb explain the polyuria (14). Papillary blood flow is not increased during cisplatin-induced polyuria, and thus can not explain the loss of medullary hypertonicity (17). Taken together, these data indicate diminished fluid reabsorption either in deeper nephrons, not accessible to micropuncture, or in the collecting ducts of cisplatin-treated animals. It is important to point out, however, that the collecting ducts are morphologically normal, suggesting the presence of an inhibitor of water transport.

Extensive necrosis of the S3, or terminal, segment of the proximal tubule is the most prominent morphological feature of cisplatin-induced renal failure (14). The reason for the special sensitivity of this nephron segment to cisplatin has not been determined, but mercury, uranyl nitrate and ischemia-induced damage show a similar cellular specificity.

C. <u>Studies on the mechanism of renal cytotoxicity</u>

We have studied several suspected targets of pathogenetic importance in cisplatin nephrotoxicity; renal cell respiration and DNA. Inhibition of renal energy metabolism has been implicated in the nephrotoxicity of other heavy metals (18).

1. Renal Cell Respiration

Oxygen consumption was measured in an isolated tubule suspension enriched in the S3 segment of the proximal tubule under the following conditions: 1) Basal O_2 consumption in the presence of available substrates (glucose, alanine, lactate, and butyrate); 2) Uncoupled rates of respiration in the presence of 10 uM carbonyl-cyanide-m-chlorophenyl hydrazone (CCCIP); and 3) Respiration after the addition of the ionophore nystatin, 40 ug/mg protein. Nystatin, by increasing cell membrane permeability to sodium and potassium raises intracellular sodium concentration and stimulates Na/K pump activity, increases ADP generation and thus stimulates mitochondrial respiration. These studies were performed in tubules from control rats exposed to cisplatin (10^{-5} to 10^{-3} M) and transplatin (10^{-5} to 10^{-3} M) in vitro, as well as in tubules from rats given 5 mg/kg cisplatin and sacrificed 12h to 6 days later. Advantages of the enriched tubule suspension, in contradistinction to the study of isolated organelles alone, is that the normal interrelationship between the plasma membrane ion pumps and tubule oxygen consumption can be explored and intracellular organelles are exposed to the toxin after its passage through the plasma membrane and subsequent biotransformation.

In vitro incubation of normal tubules with cisplatin inhibited basal and stimulated rates of oxygen consumption at very high concentrations (10^{-3}M) only. Transplatin, which is neither antineoplastic nor nephrotoxic, but also binds to DNA and protein, decreased respiration at lower concentrations (10^{-4}M) and was a more potent inhibitor of respiration than cis-platin. In tubules isolated from rats given a nephrotoxic dose of cisplatin up to 4 days after cisplatin, a time when plasma urea concentration is already elevated, basal and stimulated rates of respiration were normal. The results of these studies would seem to indicate that neither the renal cell mitochondria nor the membrane associated Na-K ATPase are important early pathogenetic targets of cisplatin.

2. DNA Studies

There is convincing evidence that the primary biochemical lesion induced by cisplatin in cancer cells is inhibition of DNA synthesis (19,20). The inhibition of DNA synthesis is persistent and occurs at much lower doses than that necessary to inhibit RNA and protein synthesis (19). Cisplatin binds to two sites in DNA (21) inducing DNA inter- and intrastrand as well as DNA-protein crosslinks (22,23). Such bidentate binding is responsible for inhibition of DNA template replication in mammalian cells (24). Crosslinks correlate with toxicity and mutagenicity and intrastrand crosslinks are not formed by the inactive transisomer, transplatin (tDDP). DNA crosslinks increase with time after the drug is removed and they are repaired slowly (25). By contrast, tDDP forms crosslinks that are quickly removed by reparative processes within the cell (25). We therefore, wanted to determine the effect of cisplatin on DNA synthesis in renal cells.

The results of studies on DNA turnover are summarized in Figure 1. DNA turnover (specific activity of ^{3}H-thymidine in DNA one hour after the injection of the radiolabel) was examined in tissue from the outer cortex and the outer stripe of the outer medulla 1, 2, 3, 4, and 7 days after cisplatin at a dose of 5 mg/kg.

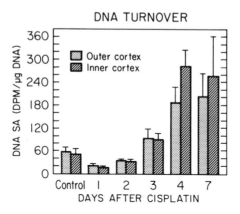

Figure 1. ^{3}H-Thymidine (1.0 uCi/g body weight) was injected intraperitoneally 1 hour prior to sacrifice and the kidneys were removed, decapsulated, weighed and homogenized in 3 volumes of ice-cold buffer consisting of 10mM Tris, pH 7.4, 1.0% Triton X-100, and 10 mM EDTA. DNA was extracted by the method of Munro and Fleck (26).[3]H activity in DNA extracts was determined in a liquid scintillation spectrometer (Packard Tri-Carb model 2425, Downers Grove IL) and DNA concentration was analyzed by the indole method as described by Ceriotti (27). Counting was carried out to at least 5000 cpm. The data is expressed as DPM/ug DNA using external quench correction. Protein was determined by the method of Lowry et. al.(28).

The specific activity of ^{3}H-thymidine in renal DNA declined significantly 1 day after the injection of cisplatin. By day 3, thymidine incorporation into renal DNA had returned to control levels and by day 7 was nearly 5 times greater than control.

The inhibition of renal DNA replication is reminiscent of cisplatin's effect on tumor and normal cells in culture and suggests that renal DNA is damaged by cisplatin. It is of interest that both the outer cortex and outer stripe of the outer medulla have reduced DNA synthesis one day after cisplatin since only the proximal tubule cells of the outer stripe undergo necrosis. At least three possibilities may be considered. First, inhibition of DNA synthesis may be irrelevant to the cytotoxicity. That it occurs so early after exposure to cisplatin and the importance of DNA synthesis inhibition to cisplatin cytotoxicity in other cells seem inconsistent with that notion. Second, cells of the outer cortex repair their DNA lesions while those of the pars recta cannot. Studies in cells whose repair processes are deficient show that cisplatin is especially toxic in them (29) making such a possibility likely. Third, it may be that the levels of the DNA adducts formed in the pars recta cells are lethal while lower levels in the earlier proximal segments are not. Further studies will be necessary to determine the importance of this observation.

The phenomenon of the higher DNA turnover, which occurs throughout the cortex and outer stripe of the outer medulla, is harder to explain. Increased DNA turnover in the outer stripe region probably reflects new and rapidly regenerating cells that replace the cells lost from this region due to cisplatin, as is usually observed after nephrotoxic insult. The increase in DNA turnover in the outer cortex, however, does not follow cell necrosis. Such stimulation of DNA synthesis in regions of the kidney unassociated with damge after nephrotoxic injury occurs in many other forms of ARF, including mercuric chloride and aminoglycoside damage (30,31). This general stimulation of renal DNA synthesis is consistent with the notion that growth factors may be released into the urine in response to injury and affect cells elsewhere in the kidney (32).

Because the increase in the thymidine incorporation into DNA occured in regions of the kidney that were not undergoing cellular necrosis, we performed autoradiographic studies to determine what specific cells are involved in increased DNA synthesis. We studied animals sacrificed 5 days after cisplatin treatment, since renal failure, cell necrosis, and renal regeneration are all well established at this time. The number of labelled specific cell nuclei (more than 4 grains per nucleus) per high powered (100X) field in control animals, was very low and never exceeded more than one nucleus for any cell type. Plate 1 shows the labeling seen in the superficial cortex of cisplatin-treated (A) and control (B) animals. On average, 10 cells/hpf were labelled in the outer cortex of cisplatin-treated animals, with distal tubules and interstitial cells (4 each) comprising the majority of labelled cells.

An average of 145 cells/hpf were labelled in the outer stripe of the outer medulla (Plate 2). Two-thirds of the cells were lining tubules whose lumens were filled with necrotic cells and most likely represent cells replacing necrotic proximal pars recta cells. The remaining cells were interstitial or endothelial cells. Cells in the inner medulla (Plate 3) were also labelled and the majority of these cells were collecting duct and interstitial cells. We also observed labelling of urothelial and interstitial cells along the papilla as well.

These initial autoradiographic studies confirm the stimulation of DNA synthesis in regions of the kidney outside the area of necrosis. Epithelial cells distal to the damaged area of the nephron, including the cells of the urothelium, as well as cells outside the tubule compartment, were labelled suggesting that a factor or factors, may be released into the tubular fluid that stimulate DNA synthesis in cells further down the nephron. Similar stimulation of cell proliferation outside the area of necrosis has been observed after other forms of nephrotoxic damage (33,34) suggesting that these observations are not unique to cisplatin.

As it was possible that growth factors were released into the tubule fluid during cisplatin-induced nephrotoxic damage, a series of experiments were initiated to determine if the expression of proto-oncogenes was increased during cisplatin-induced renal failure. That such proto-oncogenes may play a role in kidney regeneration is suggested by studies that demonstrate the existence of receptors for EGF and PDGF in mesangial, proximal, distal tubule, and collecting duct cells (35-37). EGF and PDGF stimulate DNA synthesis in these cells when added to their growth media (35-37). Furthermore, increased c-myc expression has been recently reported after folate administration to mice (38). These studies strongly suggest that renal cell proliferation may be regulated by proto-oncogenes, and/or related growth factors.

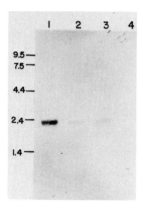

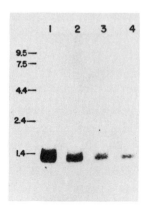

Figure 2   Figure 3

Figure 2 and 3. Northern blots of renal cortical polyadenylated RNA [poly(A)$^+$RNA] was isolated from rats, 2 and 3 days after cisplatin treatment, and hybridized to ^{32}P-labelled v-onc DNA probes (Sp. Act 5 x 10^8 cpm/ug DNA) prepared by nick-translation of v-Ha-ras (figure 2) and v-fos (figure 3) sequences isolated from plasmids HB-11 (39) and pfos-1 (40), respectively. Both plasmid were obtained from American Type Culture Collection (Rockville, MD). RNA isolated from rat kidney 2 days after cisplatin (lane 1) or vehicle treatment (lane 2). RNA isolated from rat kidney 3 days after cisplatin (lane 3) or vehicle treatment (lane 4).

The results show that in both cases, the RNA isolated 2 days after cisplatin injection, contains significantly more specific proto-oncogene transcripts than non-induced control (lanes 1 and 2 respectively). This dramatic difference disappears on day 3 post injection when levels of both transcripts are similar in induced and uninduced tissue (lanes 3 and 4). Both c-fos (fig. 2) and c-Ha-ras (fig. 3) expression were elevated when renal function was normal (BUN 17) and decreased (returned to normal levels) by the third day, when renal function declined (BUN 40). Also the expression of these proto-oncogenes was elevated before the peak of the ^{3}H-thymidine incorporation that was noted in the previous studies (see above). The sizes of the detected transcripts are approximately 1.4 and 2.3 kb for c-Ha-ras and c- fos, respectively, which is in close agreement with previously reported data (41). Normal levels of expression, with respect to control, of c-myc, c-sis and c-erb B genes, at the same time periods post cisplatin injection, were also found (data not shown). Therefore, it seems that specific proto-oncogenes are expressed before the onset of renal failure and renal regeneration. It would be interesting to determine if other proto-oncogenes are expressed at earlier and later time periods during the course of cisplatin-induced nephrotoxicity. Also, as only certain genes undergo such rapid changes in the level of their expression, these studies suggest that the regenerative response to a nephrotoxin is highly regulated.

D. A Proposed Mechanism for Cisplatin-induced Renal Failure.

The temporal sequence in renal DNA synthesis, polyuria, and reduced GFR after a single 5 mg/kg dose of cisplatin is shown in figure 4.

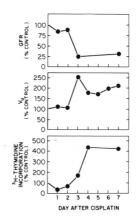

Figure 4

Enhanced renal thymidine incorporation is contemporaneous with the fall in GFR and polyuria, suggesting a possible link between them. The temporal relationship of enhanced renal DNA synthesis, accelerated cell mitosis and regeneration, and reduced GFR is also characteristic of mercury chloride, folic acid and gentamicin-induced ARF (35,42,43). Could there be a causal relationship between cell necrosis, the process of repair and regeneration, and the hemodynamic and reabsorptive events that give rise to the syndrome of acute renal failure?

Less obvious than their role in renal regeneration perhaps is their potential role in the physiologic abnormalities that characterize acute renal failure after cellular injury. Because the intracellular signals produced by EGF, type-beta transforming growth factor (TGFbeta), and PDGF are similar to those produced by vasocontrictor hormones such as vasopressin and angiotensin II (44-47), it is not suprising to discover that EGF induces constriction of aortic smooth muscle (47). Its potential role in

the altered vascular reactivity of atherosclerotic vascular
disease is, at the present time, an area of active research. Very
recent work shows that mesangial cells synthesize platelet
derived growth factor (48) and contract after exposure to it
(46). As these cells are thought to regulate glomerular filtration rate (GFR) by their state of contraction (50), it is
possible that the synthesis of a growth factor with vasoconstric-
tive properties produced during the process of regeneration, and
limited in its production to the kidney, is responsible for the
glomerular microvascular changes that underlie the fall in GFR in
acute renal failure (51, 52). The similarities in these intracellular events, and those produced by hormones known to affect
salt and water transport, also raise the possiblity that they may
be involved in the salt and water transport abnormalities that
characterize acute renal failure.

Figure 5 then outlines a proposed scheme of nephrotoxic renal failure that incorporates the features already described.

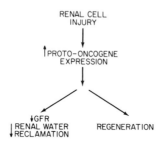

Figure 5

Renal cell injury provoked by cisplatin increases the expression of proto-oncogenes and other genes regulating cell replication. The products of some of these genes modifies the function of other cells within the kidney, such as vascular smooth muscle and tubule epithelial cells, so that the physiologic consequences of renal cell injury, high renal vascular resistance, reduced glomerular filtration and reduced water reclamation, are expressed along with the proliferative phenotype. An understanding of which factors are produced at various stages of ARF, how their synthesis is regulated both at the transcriptional and translational level, what cells are involved in their expression, and how they might effect renal function is likely to yield meaningful new insights into the specific problem of cisplatin-induced renal failure as well as provide new insights into the problem of nephrotoxic renal failure.

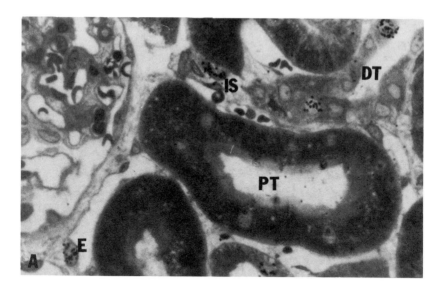

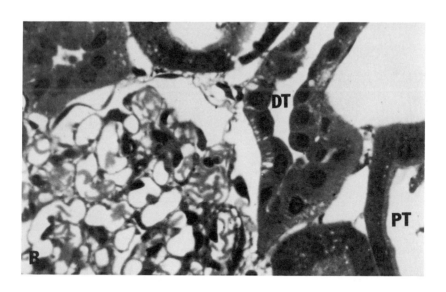

Plate 1. Representative photomicrographs of superficial cortical tissue from control (B) and cisplatin-treated (A) rats. Silver grains are infrequently seen in the control slides and show a random distribution over cell organelles. In sections of the cisplatin-treated animal, however, many grains overly nucleii of distal tubule (DT), interstitial (IS) and endothelial (E) cells. Proximal convoluted tubule (PT) cells contain no grains.

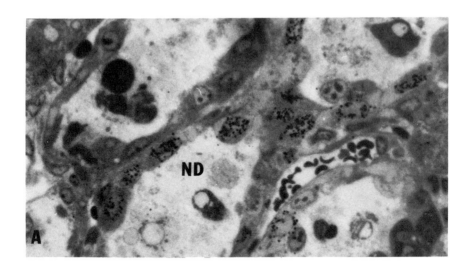

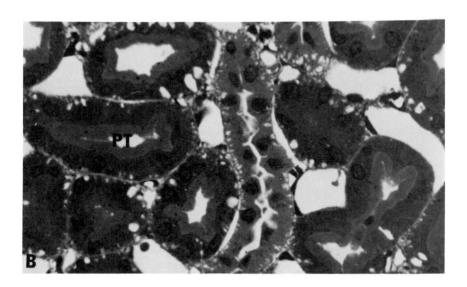

Plate 2. Photomicrographs of sections from the outer stripe of the
outer medulla. Again a random distribution of silver grains is seen
in control sections (B). Intense staining of many of the cell
nucleii that line tubules filled with necrotic debris (ND) can be seen
in the sections of the cisplatin-treated animals.

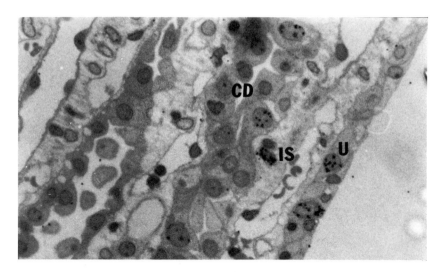

Plate 3. Photomicrograph of the inner medullary region adjacent to the renal calyx of a cisplatin-treated animal. Very low background grain density was apparent in the control section from this region. Numerous silver grains can be seen over nucleii of collecting duct (CD), interstitial (IS), and urothelial (U) cells.

REFERENCES

1. Meijer S, Mulder NH, Sleijfer DT, et al. Pharmacol. 8:27-30, 1982.
2. Goldstein MH, Safirstein R. Abstracts, 8th International Congress of Nephrology, June 1981, p.229.
3. Yuhas JM, Culo F. Cancer Treat Rep 64: 57-64, 1980.
4. Borch RF, Pleasants ME. Proc. Natl. Acad. Sci USA 76:6611-6614, 1979.
5. Berry J-P, Pauwells C, Tlouzeau S, Lespinats G. Cancer Research 44: 2864-2868, 1984.
6. Litterst CL, Torres IJ, Guarino AM. J. Clin. Hemat. and Oncol.7:169-178, 1977.
7. Safirstein R, Daye M, Miller P, Guttenplan J. Fed. Proc. 40:651A, 1980.
8. Safirstein R, Miller P, Guttenplan JB. Kidney Int. 25: 753-758, 1984.
9. Jacobs C, Kalman SM, Tretton M, Weiner MW. Cancer Treat. Rep. 64: 1223-1226, 1980.
10. Levi J, Jacobs C, Kalman S, McTigue M, Weiner MW. J. Pharmacol. Exp. Ther 213:545-550,1980.
11. Safirstein R, Winston J, Moel D, Dikman S, Guttenplan J. Int. J. Androl 10:325-245, 1987
12. Safirstein RL, Daye M, Guttenplan JB. Cancer Letters 18:329-338, 1983.
13. Lecointe P, MacQuet J-P, Butone J-L. Biochem. Biophys. Res. Comm. 90: 209-213, 1979.
14. Safirstein R, Miller P, Dikman S, Lyman N, Shapiro C. Am. J. Physiol: 241 (Renal Fluid Electrolyte Physiol. 10): F175-F185, 1982.
15. Winston J, Safirstein R. Amer. J. Physiol. 249 (Renal Fluid Electrolyte Physiol.18): F490-F496, 1985.
16. Clifton G, Pearce C, O'Neill W, Shah S, Wallin J. Clin Res. 28: 655A, 1980.
17. Safirstein R, Miller P, Dikman S. In:Acute Renal Failure, Eliahou HE ed., Libbey, London, pp 91-95, 1982.
18. Humes HD, Weinberg JM. In: Acute Renal Failure, eds Brenner BM, Lazarus JM, Phila., Saunders WB, 1983, pp 47-98.
19. Harder HC, Rosenberg B. Int. J. Cancer 6:207-216, 1970;
20. Howle JA, Gale GR. Biochem. Pharmacol. 19; 2757-2762,1970.
21. Munchausen LL, Rahn RO. Cancer Chemother. Rep. 59:643-646,1975.
22. Roberts JJ, Prascoe JM Nature 235:282-284,1972.
23. Zwelling LA, Anderson T, Kohn KW. Cancer Res. 39:365-369,1979.
24. Harder HC,Smith RG, LeRoy A Proc. Amer Assoc Cancer Research 17:80,   1976.
25. Plooy ACM, van Dijk M, Lohman PH. Cancer Research 44: 2043-2051, 1984.
26. Munro HN, Fleck A. Methods In Biochemical Analysis. Ed. D. Gloick, New York, John Wiley and Sons 1966, V14, pp.113-176.
27. Ceriotti G. J. Biol. Chem. 198: 297-303, 1952.
28. Lowry OH, Rosebrough NJ, Farr AL, Randall RJ. J. Biol. Chem. 193: 265-268, 1951.

29. Fraval HNA, Rawlings CJ, Roberts JJ, Mutat. Res. 51:121-132, 1978

30. Threlfall G, Taylor DM, Buck AT.   Lab Invest. 15: 1477-1485, 1966.

31. Laurent G, Maldague P, Carlier M, Tulkens PM.   Antimicrob Agents Chemother 24: 586-593, 1983.

32. Toback FG. Control of renal regeneration after acute tubule necrosis. In Nephrology, Robinson RR ed.,Springer-Verlag, New York, Berlin, Heidelberg, Tokyo, 1984, pp 748-762.

33. Oliver J. Am J Med 15: 535-559, 1953

34. Haagsma BH, Pound AW. Br. J. Exp Pathol 61:229-241, 1980

35. Tsivitse P, Abboud HE, Saunders C, Krauss TC.   Kidney Int. 31: 184A, 1987.

36. Stanton RC, Seifter JL.   IBID 182A.

37. Boyer DC, Stanton RC, Seifter JL.   IBID 161A.

38. Cowley BD Jr, Smardo FL Jr, Grantham JJ, Calvert JP. Kidney

39. Ellis RW, DeFeo D, Shih TY, Gonda MA, Young HA, Tsuchida N, Lowy DR, Scolnick EM. Nature 292: 506-511, 1981

40. Curran T, Peters G, von Beveren C, Teich NM, Verma IM. J. Virol. 44: 674-682, 1982

41. Muller R, Slamon DJ, Tremblay JN, Cline MJ, Verma IM. Nature

42. Bishop JM.   Ann. Rev. Biochem 52: 301-354, 1983.

43. Goyette M, Petropoulos CJ, Shank PR, Fausto N.   Science 219: 510-512, 1983.
    Int.31:163A, 1987

44. Marx JL.   Science 224: 271-274, 1984.

45. Exton JH.   J. Clin. Invest. 75: 1753-1757, 1985.

46. Berridge MJ.   Biochem J. 220: 345-360, 1984.

47. Berk BC, Brock TA, Webb RC, Taubman MB, Atkinson WJ, Gimbrone MA, Jr., Alexander RW.   J. Clin. Invest. 75: 1083-1086,   1985.

48. Mene P, Abboud HE, Dubyak GR, DiCorleto P, Scarpa A, Dunn MJ.Kidney Int. 31: 175A, 1987.

49. Abboud HE, DiCorleto P, Shultz P, Poptic E, Silver B. Kidney Int. 31: 158A, 1987.

50. Schor N, Ichikawa I, Brenner BM.   Kidney Int. 20: 442-451, 1981.

51. Baylis C, Rennke HR, Brenner BM.   Kidney Int. 12: 344-353, 1977.

52. Blantz RC.   J. Clin. Invest 55: 621-635, 1975. 299: 640-644, 1982

Experimental Approaches to Reducing Platinum Induced Kidney Toxicity

R.F. Borch, P.C. Dedon, and T.J. Montine

INTRODUCTION

The kidney is the critical organ involved with cisplatin (DDP) pharmacology; it plays a major role in drug excretion, in platinum accumulation, and it represents the primary target for dose-limiting toxicity (1). Numerous strategies have been developed to reduce this toxicity. Hydration-diuresis regimens are now a standard component in most clinical protocols, and pharmacologic approaches designed to alter renal transport or accumulation of cisplatin or its toxic metabolites have also been explored. More recently, attention has focused on the development of agents that will react with and inactivate the toxic species involved. Most of these chemoprotectors contain a nucleophilic sulfur moiety, based upon the high affinity of sulfur containing ligands for platinum complexes. However, the reaction of platinum drugs or their metabolites may also inhibit the cytotoxic reaction in the tumor cell, thus diminishing the antitumor effect. Currently the most promising inhibitors of cisplatin-induced nephrotoxicity are WR-2721, thiosulfate, and diethyldithiocarbamate (DDTC). These agents are anionic, hydrophilic, and either possess or can generate a highly reactive sulfur nucleophile (Fig. 1). All three drugs can be administered under conditions where nephrotoxicity is diminished without apparent reduction in antitumor effect. Several factors may contribute to this selectivity. First, selective concentration of the chemoprotector may occur in normal vs. tumor cells. Yuhas has suggested that drug hydrophilicity may be the major factor in the preferential concentration of WR-2721 in normal tissues vs. tumor cells (2). Concentration of these agents in proximal tubule cells via anion transport may be especially important in the kidney. Second, differences in timing or route of administration may favor inactivation of reactive metabolites in susceptible host tissues. Third, fundamental differences in chemoprotector reaction rates with tumor toxic vs. host toxic platinum complexes might reverse the toxic lesions in normal tissue without altering the presumed cytotoxic platinum-DNA complex in the tumor cell (3). Although the structural similarities of these agents are apparent, it is likely that their mechanisms of action and their potential for protection of other tissues are very different. Additional mechanistic and in vitro studies from our laboratory provide further support for this hypothesis.

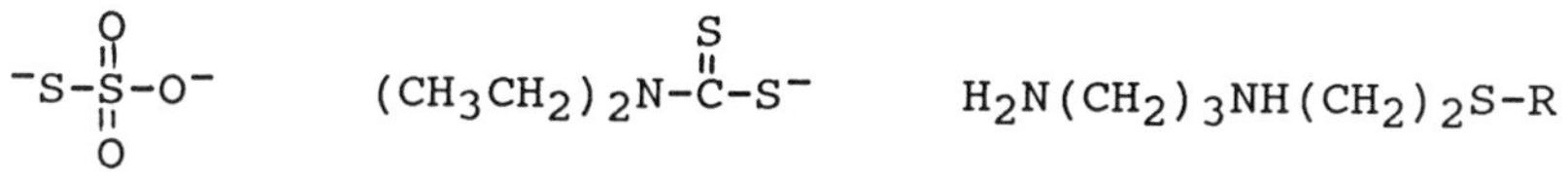

$$^-S-\overset{\overset{\displaystyle O}{\|}}{\underset{\underset{\displaystyle O}{\|}}{S}}-O^- \qquad (CH_3CH_2)_2N-\overset{\overset{\displaystyle S}{\|}}{C}-S^- \qquad H_2N(CH_2)_3NH(CH_2)_2S-R$$

A   **B**   **C,** $R = -P(O)(OH)_2$

                                                        D, $R = -H$

Fig. 1. Structures of cisplatin chemoprotectors. A: Thiosulfate; B: Diethyldithiocarbamate; C: WR-2721; D: WR-1065.

CHEMISTRY

The biologic activity of the platinum antitumor agents is governed by ligand exchange reactions with a variety of nucleophiles. For nucleophiles of low reactivity, reaction occurs via first-order rate-limiting displacement of chloride or carboxylate by water; subsequent exchange of water and nucleophile lead to rapid formation of product. For the more reactive sulfur nucleophiles, a second-order reaction involving direct displacement of the chloride or carboxylate ligand can also occur; the rate of the direct reaction will be dependent upon nucleophile concentration and will generally be competitive with the two-step process only for thiol concentrations in the millimolar range.

Table 1. Second-order rate constants and estimated half-times for platinum complex substitution reactions (pH 7.4, 37°) (adapted from ref. 3)

Reactants	$k_2 \times 10^4$ $(M-s)^{-1}$	$t_{1/2}$ (min)[a]
CISPLATIN		
Water	0.02	105 (55 M)
Glutathione	132	174 (5 mM)
Thiosulfate	570	202 (1 mM), 10 (20 mM)
DDTC	614	187 (1 mM)
CARBOPLATIN		
Water	0.00018	11,500 (55 M)
Glutathione	9.2	2500 (5 mM)
Thiosulfate	85	1350 (1 mM), 68 (20mM)
DDTC	76	1510 (1 mM)
IPROPLATIN		
Water	0.0007	2960 (55 M)
Glutathione	6.0	3800 (5 mM)
DDTC	6.6	17,400 (1 mM)
TRANS-DDP		
Water	0.074	28 (55 M)
Glutathione	39,100	0.59 (5 mM)
DDTC	255,000	0.45 (1 mM)
Pt(GSH)$_2$		
Thiosulfate	< 1	> 10^6 (1 mM)
DDTC	499	230 (1 mM)

[a] nucleophile concentration in parentheses.

In order to assess the importance of platinum - thiol reaction rates to chemoprotector efficacy, the kinetics of several platinum complexes and thiols were measured. WR-2721 was excluded because of the ambiguities surrounding transport and thiophosphate hydrolysis in vivo. The second-order rate constants and the estimated reaction half-times at physiologic or pharmacologic nucleophile concentrations are summarized in Table 1. These rate constants vary over many orders of magnitude and clearly depend on both the ligand substitution and geometry of the platinum complex and the structure of the nucleophile. Thiols react 300-400 fold faster with trans-DDP than with cisplatin and 7-14 fold faster with cisplatin than with carboplatin. DDTC is 5-8 fold more reactive than glutathione (GSH) with the Pt(II) complexes. The short half-time for reaction of trans-DDP with GSH (< 1 min @ 5 mM GSH) may account for the rapid inactivation of this platinum complex. It is interesting to note that DDTC and thiosulfate react at comparable rates with cisplatin and carboplatin. The half-times of 3 and 24 hr with cisplatin and carboplatin, respectively, suggest that, in the absence of a specific concentrating mechanism, the reaction of both DDTC and thiosulfate with the platinum drugs is too slow to be biologically significant. In contrast, DDTC and thiosulfate differ markedly in their abilities to chelate platinum bound to a thiol ligand. DDTC reacts with the cisplatin-GSH complex at a rate comparable to that for reaction with cisplatin, but thiosulfate is essentially unreactive toward this complex. Similarly, DDTC treatment restores the enzyme activity of cisplatin-inhibited rat kidney g-glutamyl transpeptidase (GGT) in vitro; thiosulfate has no effect on the inhibited enzyme (Fig. 2) (3).

The platinum drugs react very slowly with GSH at typical intracellular concentrations; the fastest reaction (cisplatin + 5 mM GSH) has a half-time of almost 3 hr. Although it has been suggested that elevated levels of intracellular GSH contribute to decreased platinum drug toxicity in normal cells and to increased drug resistance in tumor cells, it is unlikely that this involves a direct reaction between GSH and parent drug. However,

GSH may reduce cytotoxicity by rapid reaction and inactivation of aquated platinum complexes or other intracellular metabolites. The rate of cisplatin binding to salmon testes (ST) DNA decreased to 25% of control in the presence of 5 mM GSH (Fig. 3), suggesting that GSH effectively competes with DNA for reactive platinum intermediates. Platinum-DNA binding was not observed when ST DNA was treated with the preformed cisplatin-GSH complex.

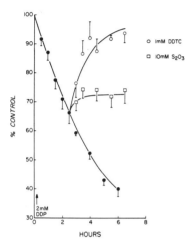

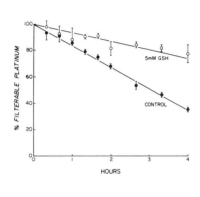

Fig. 2. Inhibition of rat GGT by 2 mM DDP (●) and reactivation by DDTC (○) or thiosulfate (□).

Fig. 3. Inhibition of DDP binding to salmon testes DNA by glutathione (5 mM).

IN VITRO STUDIES WITH LLC-PK1 CELL LINE

Our hypothesis regarding the unique property of DDTC to rescue normal tissues from platinum drug toxicity is based upon DDTC's ability to remove platinum from binding sites other than guanine bases in DNA (4,5). This hypothesis implies that either 1) DNA is not the cytotoxic target in normal cells, or 2) if DNA is the target, the platinum drug has not formed a bidentate chelate with guanine at the time of DDTC treatment. We have initiated experiments using the LLC-PK1 cell line as an in vitro model for studying the mechanistic basis of cisplatin nephrotoxicity and DDTC amelioration. LLC-PK1 is an immortal epithelial cell line derived from porcine kidney that, when grown to a confluent monolayer, expresses many functions characteristic of proximal tubule cells (6). Cell viability measured by lactate dehydrogenase activity or by total protein adherent to the culture plate gave consistent and identical results which were confirmed by trypan blue exclusion. Viability of LLC-PK1 monolayers treated with cisplatin (200-400 uM, 1 hr) was > 95% and > 90% 2 and 12 hours after treatment, respectively. Viability decreased in a dose- and time-dependent manner after 12 hours; at 72 hours, viability had decreased to 71, 35, and 10% of control, respectively, following 1-hr treatment with 200, 300, and 400 uM cisplatin (Fig. 4). One-hour treatment with the non-nephrotoxic analogs carboplatin and iproplatin caused no loss of viability at concentrations up to 2 mM. Trans-DDP (2 mM, 1 hr) reduced viability to 52%, suggesting that it is 5-10 fold less toxic than cisplatin. Toxicity appears to be dependent upon drug intensity; decreases in viability were essentially identical when cells were treated at 800 uM for 30 min and 400 uM for 60 min (14 vs. 10%), or at 600 uM for 30 min and 300 uM for 60 min (33 vs. 35%).

DDTC and thiosulfate significantly increase the viability of cisplatin-treated cells, and the time dependence of thiosulfate protection is essentially identical to that observed in vivo (7). When the monolayer is washed and then treated with DDTC (1 mM for 1 hr), significant increases in 72-hr viability are observed at all cisplatin concentrations (Fig. 4). Viability after treatment with 3 mM DDTC was marginally greater than with 1 mM DDTC (97, 85, and 42% vs. 86, 72, and 34% at 200, 300, and 400 uM cisplatin, respectively). It is interesting to note that pretreatment with DDTC is at least as effective as posttreatment in improving cell viability (Fig. 4). Pretreatment with thiosulfate (1 mM, 1 hr) afforded the best viability of any cisplatin-treated group (Fig. 5). However, thiosulfate had no effect on viability when used after cisplatin, in accord with the in vivo results. Thus it appears that both DDTC and thiosulfate enter the LLC-PK1 cells, and both decrease cisplatin toxicity when treatment occurs just prior to cisplatin exposure. Given the similar physical properties and chemical reactivity of thiosulfate and DDTC toward reactive

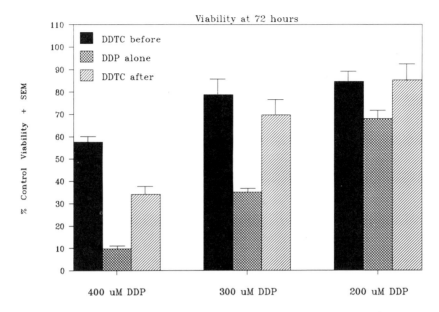

Fig. 4. Viability of LLC-PK1 cells after treatment with cisplatin (200-400 uM, 60 min) with or without DDTC (1 mM, 60 min) before or after cisplatin. Viability measured 72 hr after cisplatin treatment.

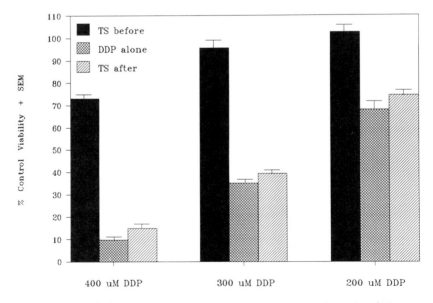

Fig. 5. Viability of LLC-PK1 cells after treatment with cisplatin (200-400 uM, 60 min) with or without thiosulfate (1 mM, 60 min) before or after cisplatin. Viability measured 72 hr after cisplatin treatment.

platinum complexes, this result is not surprising. DDTC is uniquely able to diminish cisplatin toxicity when given after cisplatin treatment. We have measured total platinum and the platinum-DDTC complex separately in these cells using AAS and HPLC assays, respectively. Intracellular platinum concentrations were 120 and 190 uM following 1-hr treatment with 200 and 400 uM cisplatin, respectively; identical platinum concentrations were found after washing the cells and then treating with DDTC (3 mM, 1 hr). Extraction of the cells and analysis of $Pt(DDTC)_2$ by HPLC showed that the DDTC chelate represents 10-20% of the platinum in the DDTC-treated cells.

THE BASIS FOR CHEMOPROTECTOR SELECTIVITY
WR-2721

The mechanistic basis for WR-2721 selectivity is not fully understood. Yuhas has shown that WR-2721 is differentially absorbed in normal and tumor cells, and that the presence of the hydrophilic thiophosphate moiety is essential for this differential uptake to occur (2). The protective effects of WR-2721 presumably require hydrolysis of the thiophosphate ester to generate the free thiol (WR-1065); this compound is a diaminothiol and should be a potent tridentate chelating agent. In contrast to the parent thiophosphate, WR-1065 shows no selectivity in its uptake in normal vs. tumor cells (2). WR-1065 has been shown to inhibit cisplatin cytotoxicity in V79 cells in vitro (8), but the results of clinical trials suggest that WR-2721 does not protect against the antineoplastic effects of cisplatin (9). WR-2721 is effective when administered just prior to cisplatin. These data are consistent with a mechanism involving WR-2721 acting as a prodrug to deliver WR-1065 selectively to normal vs. tumor cells. WR-1065 is present in the cells at the time of cisplatin administration and presumably chelates toxic platinum metabolites as they are formed. Selectivity is presumably based upon tissue distribution of WR-1065 rather than on chemical specificity, so that any cells that accumulate sufficient concentrations of thiol should be protected.

Thiosulfate

Thiosulfate reduces cisplatin-induced nephrotoxicity only when administered just prior to or concurrent with cisplatin administration (10). It has no effect on other systemic toxicities associated with cisplatin administration, and it is ineffective when given after cisplatin. Thiosulfate does not alter plasma or renal distribution of platinum (11), it does not restore activity to cisplatin-inhibited enzymes (3), and its rate of reaction with cisplatin at pharmacologic plasma thiosulfate concentrations is too slow to account for protection by direct reaction with and inactivation of the parent drug. However, the anion transport system in the proximal tubule may increase the intracellular thiosulfate concentration substantially; at thiosulfate concentrations in excess of 20 mM, the half-time for inactivation of cisplatin would be < 10 minutes (see Table 1). Thus thiosulfate selectivity may result from concentration of this inorganic anion in the proximal tubule cells of the kidney; higher intracellular concentrations lead to more rapid inactivation of cisplatin or its nephrotoxic metabolites within the tubule cell.

DDTC

DDTC is unique in its ability to act as a "rescue" agent and reduce platinum drug toxicity even when administered several hours after cisplatin. It removes platinum from the kidney, restores the activity of enzymes inhibited by platinum drugs, and protects against systemic toxicities in addition to the kidney (3-5). Although the reaction kinetics of DDTC with platinum complexes are generally slow, DDTC appears to remove platinum from all biologically relevant binding sites except bis-guanine complexes in DNA (4). DDTC does not protect against platinum drug antitumor activity when administered appropriately; an interval between platinum drug and DDTC administration sufficient to allow drug binding to DNA in tumor cells should be maintained, however. Thus chemical reactivity appears to be a major component of DDTC selectivity; it is administered after the platinum drug has undergone distribution and binding to cellular targets, and it may reverse drug binding at sites other than bis-guanine cross-links in DNA.

Although the exact mechanism by which platinum drugs produce toxicity in the kidney and other tissues is not known, the effects of these chemoprotectors provide several clues. First, the toxic lesion probably forms within minutes of cisplatin exposure. Both WR-2721 and thiosulfate are protective only when present just prior to or during cisplatin treatment. Second, the DDTC experiments suggest that the toxic lesion must be reversible for at least several hours. Third, this early lesion is reversible by DDTC, implying that if DNA is the target for the toxic reaction, a DDTC-reactive platinum intermediate must be formed with a lifetime of minutes to hours. Rescue timing is even more dramatic in the bone marrow, where significant protection is observed when DDTC is given as long as 5 hours after cisplatin or carboplatin (5, 12). Finally, a major dilemma remains in that the nephrotoxic lesion must form within minutes and be reversed within several hours, but significant changes in physiology and viability don't occur until 48-72 hours (13).

CLINICAL STATUS OF PLATINUM CHEMOPROTECTORS

WR-2721, thiosulfate, and DDTC are at different stages of clinical development; both the benefits and the limitations of the first two agents are reasonably well defined, but neither has been established for DDTC. It is very difficult to establish with certainty the extent to which any of these agents alone will reduce clinical nephrotoxicity. All of the cisplatin-chemoprotector protocols also incorporate vigorous hydration/diuresis regimens, so the increase in maximum tolerated dose (MTD) of cisplatin results from the combination of chemoprotector and hydration. Recent studies also suggest that bone marrow and/or neurotoxicity are more likely to be dose-limiting at higher platinum drug doses, so a chemoprotector should also ameliorate these toxicities to achieve a significant increase in platinum drug MTD. Thiosulfate has been most impressive in protecting the kidney against cisplatin toxicity; cisplatin doses of 200 mg/m^2 with concomitant thiosulfate infusion have been administered with minimal nephrotoxicity.

Unfortunately, significant bone marrow and neurotoxicity was observed at this dose (10), suggesting that thiosulfate's specificity for protection of the kidney will limit its use at high doses of platinum drugs. Recently published clinical studies report impressive response rates and minimal toxicity with WR-2721 and cisplatin (9, 14); however, it appears that the MTD of cisplatin with WR-2721 (at its MTD of 740 mg/m^2) will be in the range of 135-150 mg/m^2. Our Phase I trial showed that DDTC is tolerated at a dose of 4 g/m^2 given as a 45-minute iv infusion (15). Pharmacokinetic studies indicate that DDTC is rapidly cleared, and that doses in this range give steady-state plasma levels and AUC values greater than those required for kidney, gut, and bone marrow protection in rodents (Table 2 and ref. 5). In cases where the DDTC infusion time was extended much beyond one

Table 2. DDTC pharmacokinetic parameters in man, rat, and mouse (n = 5)

Dose (g/m^2)	$t_{1/2}$ (min)	c_p (uM)	AUC (mM-min)	V_D (ml/kg)	Cl (ml/min-kg)
MAN[a]					
2.8	13.4	400	21	290	14.7
4.6[b]	12.2	1070	53	230	11.2
7.5[b,c]	14.9	850	46	330	13.5
RAT[d]					
250	10	1170	15		
MOUSE[e]					
250	10	400	10		

[a] iv infusion over 45 minutes.
[b] n = 2.
[c] infused over 75 minutes.
[d] iv bolus; dose in mg/kg.
[e] ip bolus; dose in mg/kg.

hour, however, optimal plasma concentrations and AUC values were not achieved. Cisplatin dose-escalation trials in combination with DDTC at 4 g/m^2 are currently under investigation.

SUMMARY

Many good strategies are currently available to protect against the nephrotoxicity of cisplatin. Appropriate combination of chemoprotectors and aggressive hydration regimens may virtually eliminate nephrotoxicity as a clinically significant problem in cisplatin chemotherapy. Acute myelosuppression and cumulative neurotoxicity are emerging as the major obstacles preventing widespread application of very high-dose platinum drug therapy. Successful development of chemoprotectors to inhibit these toxicities will be the key to major advances in the clinical efficacy of existing platinum chemotherapeutic agents.

REFERENCES

1. For a recent review see Borch, R.F. (1987) In:
    Metabolism and Action of Anti-cancer Drugs eds. Prough,
    R. and Powis, G. (Taylor and Francis, London), pp.
    163-193.
2. Yuhas, J.M., Davis, M.E., Glover, D., Brown, D., Ritter,
    M. (1982) Int. J. Radiat. Oncol. Biol. Phys. 8: 519-522;
    Yuhas, J.M. (1980) Cancer Res. 40: 1519-1524.
3. Dedon, P.C. and Borch, R.F. (1987) Biochem. Pharmacol.
    36: (in press).
4. Bodenner, D.L., Dedon, P.C., Keng, P.C. and Borch, R.F.
    (1986) Cancer Res. 46: 2745-2750.
5. Bodenner, D.L., Dedon, P.C., Keng, P.C., Katz, J.C. and
    Borch, R.F. (1986) Cancer Res. 46: 2751-2755.
6. Gstraunthaler, G. and Handler, J.S. (1987) Am. J.
    Physiol. 252: C232-238.
7. Howell, S.B. and Taetle, R. (1980) Cancer Treat. Rep.
    64: 611-616.
8. Nagy, B., Dale, P.J. and Grdina, D.J. (1986) Cancer Tes.
    46 1132-1135.
9. Glover, D., Glick, J.H., Weiler, C., Fox, K. and Guerry,
    D. (1987) J. Clin. Oncol. 5: 574-578.
10. Pfeifle, C.E., Howell, S.B., Felthouse, R.D., Woliver,
    T.B.S., Andrews, P.A., Markman, M. and Murphy, M.P.
    (1985) J. Clin. Oncol. 3: 237-244.
11. Uozumi, J. and Litterst, C.L. (1985) Cancer Chemother.
    Pharmacol. 15: 93-99.
12. Gringeri, A. and Borch, R.F. (1987) Proc. Am. Assoc.
    Cancer Res. 28: 448; ibid. 25: 371.
13. Winston, J.A. and Safirstein, R. (1985) Am. J. Physiol.
    249: F490-496.
14. Glover, D., Glick, J.H., Weiler, C., Fox, K., Turrisi, A.
    and Kligerman, M. (1986) Int. J. Radiation Oncol. Biol.
    Phys. 12: 1509-1512.
15. Qazi, R., Chang, A., Borch, R., Loughner, J. and Bennett,
    J.M. (1986) Proc. Am. Soc. Clin. Oncol. 5: 31.

High Dose Cisplatin with Hypertonic Saline: Toxicity and Therapeutic Results

E. Reed, M. Poirier, R.C. Young, and R.F. Ozols

INTRODUCTION

Cisplatin is among the most active agents currently available for the treatment of malignant disease. It is particularly active in ovarian and testicular cancer. In both these diseases there is substantial clinical and laboratory evidence to indicate an important dose response relationship with cisplatin. Escalations in cisplatin dose beyond 100-120 mg/m^2, however, have not been routinely possible due to the development of dose limiting nephrotoxicity. When used with standard hydration (3 L/day of normal saline) and forced diuresis, cisplatin doses of 100-120 mg/m^2 have produced an acceptable degree of nephrotoxicity. Using this approach, however, it has been demonstrated that the incidence of renal toxicity approaches 50% when the cisplatin dose is escalated to 130-140 mg/m^2 (1).

We have examined the efficacy and toxicity of high dose cisplatin administered in hypertonic saline and with maintenance of vigorous chloruresis in patients with testicular and ovarian cancer. In addition, we have also studied the effects of high dose carboplatin, a cisplatin analog without dose limiting nephrotoxicity, in patients with refractory ovarian cancer. These clinical studies have included the measurement of N7dGpG- and dApG-diammineplatinum adducts in DNA isolated from peripheral white cells and tissues of patients treated with high dose platinum regimens.

MATERIALS AND METHODS

Administration of High Dose Cisplatin and High Dose Carboplatin

Table 1 summarizes the manner in which high dose cisplatin

and high dose carboplatin have been administered in our studies.

Patient Population

Three groups of patients were treated with high dose cisplatin or carboplatin containing regimens. Phase II trials of single agent high dose cisplatin (2) or high dose carboplatin (3) were performed in previously treated ovarian cancer patients. In addition, high dose cisplatin has been combined with cyclophosphamide in the induction therapy of previously untreated patients with advanced ovarian cancer (4). In testicular cancer, high dose cisplatin has been combined with VP-16, vinblastine, and bleomycin (PVeBV), Table 2, in the treatment of poor risk advanced nonseminomatous testicular cancer patients (5).

Table 1. Administration of High Dose Cisplatin and High Dose Carboplatin

	High Dose Cisplatin	High Dose Carboplatin
Dose:	40 mg/m^2 I.V. qd x 5	400 mg/m^2 I.V. qd x 2 by continuous infusion
Vehicle:	250 ml 3% saline	D$_5$W
Hydration:	6L per day normal saline with 20 meq KCl per liter	150 ml per hour normal saline
Diuretic:	20 mg furosemide	None

Table 2. PVeBV Chemotherapy

Cisplatin (P):	40 mg/m^2 I.V. qd x 5
Vinblastine (Ve):	0.2 mg/kg I.V. on d 1
Bleomycin (B):	30 u I.V. q wk
VP-16 (V):	100 mg/m^2 I.V. qd x 5

Cycles repeated every 21 days.

Collection of Specimens for DNA Platinum Adduct Formation

Two types of specimens were collected in these studies, nucleated peripheral blood cells and organ tissues at autopsy. On the morning following completion of cisplatin or carboplatin therapy, 35-50 ml of blood was obtained by venipuncture and placed in heparinized tubes. The blood was centrifuged at 2000 rpm for 15 mintues and the "buffy coat" was aspirated and frozen at -20°C until DNA isolation. At autopsy, selected organs were sampled and tissues were frozen without preservative at -20°C until DNA isolation.

DNA Preparation and ELISA

DNA is isolated from tissue by a CsCl gradient density centrifugation method (6). DNA was quantitated by absorbance at 260 nm and dialyzed against doubly distilled water for 36 hrs. Volume was adjusted to 700 ug DNA per ml. ELISA was performed as previously reported (7), with the same volume of DNA and of assay reagents used in all control and experimental wells of the plates.

RESULTS

Previously Treated Ovarian Cancer Patients

Tables 3 and 4 summarize the results of high dose cisplatin and high dose carboplatin in previously treated ovarian cancer patients.

Table 3. Results of Administration of High-Dose Cisplatin

Response to Therapy	No. of Patients		Percent	
Overall response rate	6/19		32	
Partial response (PR)		4/19		21
Clinical complete response (CR)		2/19		11
Minor response	3/19		16	
Disease stabilization	5/19		26	
Progressive disease	5/19		26	

Table 4. Results of High-Dose Carboplatin

Response to Therapy	Number		Percent	
Overall response rate	8		27	
PR		4		13
CR (Clinical) (Median duration 7 months)*		4		13
Minor Response	3		10	
Stable disease	7		23	
Progressive disease	12		40	
Median survival (mo)				
All patients		12		
Responding patients		>21		
Progressive disease		8		

Number of patients evaluable for response, 30. Median (range) number of cycles, four (1 to 8).
*Three of the four patients who achieved a complete CR remain clinically disease-free at 8+, 10+, and 13+ months.

On the basis of the encouraging therapeutic results of high dose cisplatin in heavily treated ovarian cancer patients, a trial of high dose cisplatin together with cyclophosphamide is currently in progress at the Medicine Branch of the National Cancer Institute. In this trial, advanced ovarian cancer patients are treated with cyclophosphamide (200 mg/m^2 qd x 5) together with cisplatin (40 mg/m^2) on the same days. Patients receive 3-4 cycles of therapy and then undergo restaging evaluation including second-look laparotomy if there is no evidence of disease on clinical studies. The preliminary results of this ongoing trial have been presented (4). Eighteen patients have been treated (68% stage III and 39% stage IV), and 56% of the patients have had >2 cm disease at the time chemotherapy was initiated. The overall response rate in the first 15 evaluable patients was 73% which included clinical complete responses in 9/15 patients (60%). Eight patients had a second-look laparotomy. Six of these patients were disease-free. Median survival for all patients has not yet been reached.

High Dose Cisplatin in Testicular Cancer Patients

In a pilot study it was demonstrated that PVeBV was effective therapy in previously untreated patients with high risk testicular cancer patients. On the basis of the pilot results, a randomized trial of PVeBV vs. standard PVeB chemotherapy in high risk testicular cancer patients is currently in progress at the Medicine Branch. Preliminary results of this trial have recently been reported (8) and summarized in Table 5.

Table 5. Preliminary Results of PVeB vs PVeBV in Poor Risk Nonseminomatous Testicular Cancer

		SURVIVAL	
	CR	Overall	Disease-Free
PVeBV	30/34 (88%)	27/34 (79%)	26/34 (76%)
PVeB	12/18 (67%)	10/18 (56%)	8/18 (44%)
2-sided p	0.14	0.14	0.03

Disease Response and DNA Platinum Adduct Formation

As we have reported (10) peak WBC adduct level correlates with disease response in a group of 25 ovarian cancer patients treated with single agent cisplatin or carboplatin chemotherapy. This group of 25 patients was a subset of the total cohort of 49 patients treated with single agent cisplatin or carboplatin therapy. Comparison of the patients studied with the total cohort of patients is shown in Table 6. As shown, the subset of the total cohort that participated in the adduct study responded to therapy at the same rate as the total cohort, suggesting that the subset studied for adduct levels reflects the biology of the total cohort. When the actual adduct values for each patient were analyzed for comparison to disease response, the two-sided p value relating adduct level to disease response was 0.018 in the high dose cisplatin group, 0.020 in the high dose carboplatin group, and 0.0015 in the total group of 25 patients. When the retrospectively chosen cut-off of 160 attomoles of adduct per ug DNA was used for stratification, this level of adduct formation in WBC DNA also correlated with disease response with a two-sided p value of 0.0013. Adduct levels have been measured in other tissues of some of the patients in these studies. As discussed below, we have begun to correlate adduct formation with drug toxicity as well.

Table 6.

Study Group	# In Clinical Study	Response Rate Clinical Study	#In Adduct Study	Response Rate Adduct Study
High Dose Cisplatin	19	32%	12	33%
High Dose Carboplatin	30	27%	13	31%
Both Groups Combined	49	29%	25	32%

Toxicity of High Dose Cisplatin

The administration of high dose cisplatin as outlined in Table 1 has essentially eliminated nephrotoxicity as the dose limiting toxicity of platinum. We have described the renal toxicity of high dose cisplatin in detail for both testicular cancer and ovarian cancer patients (2,9). In the 32% of advanced ovarian cancer patients there was a marked rise in serum creatinine (2.1 - 5.6 mg/dL) and a decreasing creatinine clearance for the first cycle of high dose cisplatin. However, renal function returned to normal in all patients over a 2-3 week period with conservative medical management. In contrast to the first cycle of high dose cisplatin, the second through fourth cycles, which were administered to the same patients who experienced renal dysfunction with the first cycle, did not produce any new apparent renal damage. Patients did not have any further elevations in serum creatinine. Over 70 advanced ovarian cancer patients have now been treated with high dose cisplatin regimens at the Medicine Branch. Only 1 patient was not able to tolerate the hydration regimen due to the development of increasing effusions. In addition, there was only 1 instance of dose modification of cisplatin in patients with advanced ovarian cancer due to the development of nephrotoxicity with the first cycle. Since we have demonstrated that these patients can be retreated with cisplatin even if they had renal dysfunction with their first cycle of therapy, we have not had to decrease the cisplatin dose because of nephrotoxicity.

In the testicular cancer patients there have been no instances of dose modification of cisplatin due to nephrotoxicity. We have administered full dose cisplatin even in patients with obstructive uropathy due to large retroperitoneal tumor masses. There was no statistically significant difference between serum creatinines and creatinine clearances pre and post 3-4 cycles of high dose cisplatin. These results should be compared to the previous reports of renal toxicity with standard dose cisplatin and standard hydration. It has been reported that there was a 40% decrease in creatinine clearance after 6 cycles of standard cisplatin dosage in patients with testicular cancer (1). These patients received the same total dose of cisplatin as the testicular cancer patients who received 3 cycles of high dose cisplatin and in the latter group of patients there was no nephrotoxicity using the schedule of administration as shown in Table 1.

The dose limiting toxicity of high dose cisplatin is neurotoxicity. Peripheral neuropathy developed in all advanced ovarian cancer patients who received more than 2 cycles of high dose cisplatin and 37% of all previously treated patients had grade III peripheral neuropathy when treated with high dose cisplatin. Initial symptoms were numbness and tingling in the distal extremities. The third and fourth cycles of high dose cisplatin were associated with even more severe neurologic toxicity. Patients frequently developed gait disturbances and/or marked difficulty in manual dexterity. This is primarily due to a profound decrease in proprioception and led 2 patients to become temporarily wheelchair dependent. In some patients, neurologic toxicity progressed even after cisplatin was stopped. It is clear that more then 3 cycles of high dose cisplatin cannot be routinely administered to patients with advanced ovarian cancer without the development of an unacceptably high rate of peripheral neuropathy. It is of particular note the patients treated with high dose carboplatin, however, did not have any neuropathy or any nephrotoxicity. The dose limiting toxicity of high dose carboplatin was the development of severe myelosuppression. The median white cell nadir was 0.6 and the median platelet nadir was 6,500 after the first cycle of high dose carboplatin. However, myelosuppression did not appear particularly cumulative (3).

Toxicities that may be Related to Platinum DNA Adduct Formation
Hematologic Toxicity

Our group has shown that adduct formation in WBC-DNA of ovarian cancer patients correlates with disease response (10). In all patients studied in our single agent high dose cisplatin (2) or high dose carboplatin (3) trials, hematologic toxicity was consistently seen. As has been noted by other investigators, hematologic toxicity appeared to be more severe in the carboplatin treated patients than in those who received cisplatin. Interestingly, peak adduct levels observed in carboplatin treated patients were consistently higher than in those patients receiving cisplatin (Table 7). Although the reason for this difference has yet to be investigated, it suggests that the esterase activity that may play a role in "activating" carboplatin to its active species (T. Bowden, E. Reed, M.C. Poirier, unpublished observations) may be present in high levels in white blood cells.

Table 7.

Patient Group	# Patients	Peak Adduct Levels Per Group: Median (Range)	Median WBC Nadir Cycle 1
High Dose Cisplatin	13	89 (0-210)	1.3
High Dose Carboplatin	12	176 (0-357)	0.6

Neurologic Toxicity

Platinum-related neurotoxicity has multiple manifestations and has been the most elusive aspect of platinum pharmacology with respect to explanatory pathophysiology (11). Various types of neurotoxicity have been related to drug-protein interactions, to possible alterations in cobalt metabolism, or have simply eluded a pathophysiologic explanation. We have repeatedly found that platinum-DNA adducts persist in several different types of nervous tissue for months following platinum chemotherapy (Table 8). These data suggest

Table 8.

Patient	Total Platinum Dose (DDP + CBDCA)	Time Since Most Recent Therapy	Nervous Tissue Studied	Adduct Level (Amol/ug DNA)
#1 (F)	1250 mg/m^2	3 wks	Brain-Gray Matter	122
			Brain-White Matter	>100
#2 (F)	7200 mg/m^2	9 mths	Brain-Gray Matter	833
			Brain-White Matter	456
			Peripheral Nerve	315

that platinum binding to DNA is substantial in Betz cells of the neurocortex, oligodendria and/or astrocytes of subcortical white matter, and Schwann cells of the peripheral nervous system. If platinum-DNA binding leads to cell death in nervous tissues as it does in other tissues, Schwann cell loss would lead to segmental demyelination which is the characteristic histologic lesion seen in platinum-related peripheral neuropathy. With most CNS illnesses, however, cell loss usually has to be severe before gross neurologic changes occur. This may be why platinum-related CNS side effects are relatively rarely observed.

Chronic Renal Dysfunction

Many studies have shown platinum-related acute renal toxicity to be related to platinum binding to proteins (12). In other studies, we have shown that acute renal dysfunction in rodents is not directly related to platinum-DNA adduct formation (C.L. Litterst, M.C. Poirier, E. Reed, unpublished observation). However, the role that adduct persistence may play in chronic renal dysfunction has yet to be defined. In the rat, platinum-DNA adduct that forms in the kidney tissue after a single I.V. exposure of drug is removed in a biphasic fashion. The initial $t_{1/2}$ is 3-4 days, followed by a more prolonged $t_{1/2}$ of greater than 14 days. In patients we have studied, two have shown platinum-related chronic renal dysfunction and at autopsy had substantive levels of platinum adduct in kidney tissue DNA (Table 9). In a third patient platinum-DNA adduct was found in

Table 9.

Patient	Time Since Most Recent Platinum Therapy	Adduct Level In Kidney Tissue DNA	Ante-Mortem Renal Function
#1 (F)	3 wks	66 attom/ug DNA	BUN 20/Creat 1.7
#2 (F)	9 mths	184 attom/ug DNA	BUN 19/Creat 0.9 Creat Cl. 42 ml/min
#3 (M)	22 mths	147 attom/ug DNA	Data not available

kidney tissue 22 months after platinum therapy, but ante-mortem data on renal function was not obtained. Although far from conclusive, these data suggest that platinum-DNA binding may be a substantive contributory factor to platinum-related chronic renal toxicity.

DISCUSSION

These results demonstrate that high dose cisplatin can be safely administered to patients with advanced ovarian cancer and testicular cancer. Using the method of administration as outlined in Table 1, high dose cisplatin does not produce dose limiting nephrotoxicity.

However, the dose limiting toxicity of high dose cisplatin now is neurotoxicity. The results in patients with advanced ovarian cancer demonstrate a high degree of activity for high dose cisplatin and high dose carboplatin. However, in the absence of a prospective randomized trial comparing high dose cisplatin vs. standard dose cisplatin therapy in previously untreated ovarian cancer patients the role of high dose therapy remains experimental. In the treatment of testicular cancer patients, it is apparent that PVeBV is superior to PVeB in the treatment of high risk patients. However, the benefit of PVeBV may relate to the double-dose cisplatin, the addition of VP-16, or to the synergistic effects of high dose cisplatin plus VP-16.

The manner in which the aggressive hydration regimen and the chloruresis protects against the nephrotoxicity of cisplatin has not been established. Our studies (Table 9) demonstrate that platinum-DNA adducts can persist in kidney tissues for extended periods of time after treatment. It is possible that DNA adduct formation in the renal tissue may contribute to platinum-related chronic toxicity.

The mechanisms responsible for cisplatin-induced neurotoxicity also remain to be established. Data in Table 8 suggest that platinum binding to DNA in Schwann cells of the peripheral nervous system may be correlated with the development of neurologic symptoms. It is clear from a clinical point of view that the incidence of neurologic toxicity markedly increases after a total dose of 600 mg/m^2 of cisplatin is administered.

Studies are in progress to determine if the dose limiting toxicities of platinum-containing compounds can be pharmacologically decreased. Clinical trials have recently been initiated at the Medicine Branch using diethyldithiocarbamate in patients receiving high dose cisplatin and high dose carboplatin. Other studies are in progress to determine whether the radioprotective agent, WR2721, can decrease the neurotoxicity of cisplatin. Finally, it is possible that colony stimulating factors which may decrease the hematologic toxicity of chemotherapeutic agents may permit even higher doses of carboplatin to be administered since the only toxicity of this agent appears to be hematologic suppression.

REFERENCES

1. Ozols RF and Young RC: High-dose cisplatin therapy in ovarian cancer. Semin Oncol 12: 21-30, 1985.
2. Ozols RF, Ostchega Y, Myers CE, and Young RC: High-dose cisplatin in hypertonic saline in refractory ovarian cancer. J Clin Oncol 3: 1246-1250, 1985.
3. Ozols RF, Ostchega, Curt G, and Young RC: High-dose carboplatin in refractory ovarian cancer patients. J Clin Oncol 5: 197-201, 1987.
4. Young RC, Myers EC, Ostchega Y, et al: CPR (cyclophosphamide, high dose cisplatin and radiation): An aggressive short term induction regimen for advanced ovarian adenocarcinoma. Proc Ann Mtg Am Soc Clin Oncol 4: 119, 1985.
5. Ozols RF, Deisseroth AB, Messerschmidt J, et al.: Treatment of poor prognosis nonseminomatous testicular cancer with a "high dose" platinum combination chemotherapy regimen. Cancer 51: 1803-1807, 1983.
6. Flamm WB, Birnstiel ML, Walker PMB. In Birnie G, and Fox SM (Eds), Subcellular Components and Fractionation. Butterworth and Co., Ltd., London. 1967; pp 129-155.
7. Reed E, Yuspa SH, Zwelling LA, Ozols RF, Poirier MC. Quantitation of cis-diamminedichloroplatinum II (cisplatin)-DNA intrastrand adducts in testicular and ovarian cancer patients receiving cisplatin chemotherapy. J Clin Inv 77, 545-550, 1986.
8. Ozols RF, Ihde D, Jacob J: Poor prognosis nonseminomatous testicular cancer: Mature results of a randomized trial of PVeBV vs PVeB. Proc Amer Soc Clin Oncol 6: 107, 1987.
9. Ozols RF, Corden BJ, Jacob J, Wesley MN, Ostchega Y, and Young RC: High-dose cisplatin in hypertonic saline. Ann Int Med 100, 19-24, 1984.
10. Reed E, Ozols RF, Tarone R, Yuspa SH, Poirier MC: Platinum-DNA adducts in leukocyte DNA correlate with disease response in ovarian cancer patients receiving platinum-based chemotherapy. Proc Natl Acad Sci USA 84, in press, 1987.
11. Reed E, Poirier MC, Katz D, Yuspa SH, Ozols RF: Formation of platinum-DNA adducts in multiple tissues of a patient with ovarian cancer: Evidence for DNA binding in neural tissues - A case report, submitted, 1987.
12. Litterst CL, Reed E: Platinum compounds. In Kaiser HE (Ed) Progressive Stages of Malignant Neoplastic Growth. Martinus Nijhoff Publishers, Norwell, Massachusetts, in press, 1987.

SECTION IV

POSTER PRESENTATIONS

POSTER PRESENTATIONS

1 EFFECT OF SODIUM CROMOGLYCATE (C) ON HISTAMINE RELEASE
AND CARDIOTOXICITY INDUCED BY EPIRUBICIN (E): *IN VITRO*
AND *IN VIVO* STUDIES
Giuliana Decorti, Fiora Bartoli Klugmann, Luigi Candussio, Sergio Bevilacqua, Franco
Mallardi, Vittorio Grill and Luciano Baldini

2 DIDOX — A NEW ANTICANCER DRUG THAT INHIBITS RIBONUCLEOTIDE
REDUCTASE, PROTECTS AGAINST TOXICITY AND POTENTIATES ANTITUMOR
ACTIVITY OF ANTHRACYCLINES
Howard Elford, Bart van't Riet and Eugene Herman

3 EFFECT OF DIFFERENT SCHEDULES OF CALCIUM ANTAGONIST AD-
MINISTRATION ON THE DOXORUBICIN INDUCED CARDIOTOXICITY IN RAT
Fabrizio Villani, Francesco Piccinini, Elena Monti, Luisa Paracchini, Luigia Favalli, An-
nalinda Rozza, Enrica Lanza and Paola Poggi

4 MECHANISM OF THE REDUCTION OF ANTHRACYCLINE ANTIBIOTICS AND
THEIR IRON COMPLEXES BY ASCORBATE: RELATIONSHIP WITH THEIR EFFECTS
ON LIPID PEROXIDATION
Igor B. Afanas'ev, Natalia I. Polozova and Vladimir I. Gunar

5 SIGNIFICANT REDUCTION OF DELAYED DOXORUBICIN CARDIOTOXICITY
BY ICRF-187 IN RATS
Luigia Favalli, Enrica Lanza, Annalinda Rozza, Paola Poggi, Milena Galimberti and
Fabrizio Villani

6 CHARACTERIZATION OF THE CARDIOPROTECTIVE EFFECT OF (S)(+)-4,4'-
PROPYLENE-2, 6-PIPERAZINEDIONE (ICRF-187) ON ANTHRACYCLINE CAR-
DIOTOXICITY
Joyce A. Filppi, Anthony R. Imondi and Richard L. Wolgemuth

7 IMMOBILIZED ADRIAMYCIN: TOXIC POTENTIAL *IN VIVO* AND *IN VITRO*
M.P. Hacker, J.S. Lazo, C.A. Pritsos and T.R. Tritton

8 DEPLETION OF POLYAMINES BY DIFLUOROMETHYLORNITHINE (DFMO)
DOES NOT ALTER DOXORUBICIN (DOX) TOXICITY
M.P. Hacker and P.J. Kimberly

9 FUNDAMENTAL STUDY OF BLEOMYCIN INDUCED PULMONARY TOXICITY
IN MICE
Hisao Ekimoto, Kimihiko Takada, Mineaki Okada, Junpei Ito, Katsutoshi Takahashi,
Akira Matsuda, Tomohisa Takita and Hamao Umezawa

10 MURINE STRAIN DIFFERENCES IN LUNG PROCOLLAGEN AND FIBRONECTIN
mRNA AFTER CONSTANT SC INFUSION OF BLEOMYCIN
Dale G. Hoyt and John S. Lazo

1 EFFECT OF SODIUM CROMOGLYCATE (C) ON HISTAMINE RELEASE AND CARDIOTOXICITY INDUCED BY EPIRUBICIN (E): "IN VITRO" AND "IN VIVO" STUDIES. Giuliana Decorti*, Fiora Bartoli Klugmann, Luigi Candussio, Sergio Bevilacqua, Franco Mallardi, Vittorio Grill and Luciano Baldini. Institute of Pharmacology, University of Trieste, Via Valerio n°32, I-34100 Trieste, ITALY.

It has recently been suggested that anthracycline associated cardiac toxicity may be mediated by the release of vasoactive substances and particularly histamine. In previous studies we have shown that adriamycin induces an important histamine release "in vitro" from rat peritoneal cells in a noncytotoxic manner. This release is very similar in its biochemical features to that induced by compound 48/80. The present study was undertaken with the aim of defining the characteristics of the release of histamine promoted by another anthracycline, E and to verify if a pretreatment with C could limit histamine release "in vitro" and "in vivo" and protect animals from the cardiomyopathy.

Rat peritoneal cells were incubated in quadruplicate with various concentrations of E; additional samples were preincubated with different concentrations of C. The amount of histamine released was assayed by a fluorimetric method. E induced an important and dose dependent histamine release at concentrations ranging from 12.5 to 100 ug/ml. This release was dependent on temperature and on intracellular calcium concentrations, was very rapid in its kinetic and was inhibited by C. Sprague Dawley rats were i.p. injected with E or E + C. Peritoneal cells were processed for microscopical examination. E induced an important degranulation of mast cells without cell disruption. No degranulation was observed in mast cells obtained from animals pretreated with C. CD1 mice were acutely (20 mg/kg) or chronically (8 mg/kg/week x 3) treated with E or E + C (200 mg/kg). Myocardial tissue was microscopically examined and lesions were quantified by means of an image analyzer Zeiss MOP Videoplan. C significantly ameliorated the survival time of animals and reduced the histopathological lesions of myocardial tissue.

These data further support the hypothesis that histamine release could play a crucial role in the pathogenesis of anthracycline cardiomyopathy and suggest a possible clinical use of C in the prevention of this side effect.

2   DIDOX - A NEW ANTICANCER DRUG THAT INHIBITS RIBONUCLEOTIDE
REDUCTASE PROTECTS AGAINST TOXICITY AND POTENTIATES ANTI-
TUMOR ACTIVITY OF ANTHRACYCLINES. Howard Elford*, Bart
van't Riet and Eugene Herman[#], Molecules for Health, Inc., 3313
Gloucester Road, Richmond, VA 23227 and [#]FDA, HFD-413, 200 "C"
Street, S.W., Washington, DC 20204.

A new series of mammalian ribonucleotide reductase inhibitors
designed to contain a polyhydroxyphenyl ring has exhibited
anticancer activity in a number of animal tumor systems. Didox
(3,4-dihydroxybenzohydroxamic acid) is the best of the first
generation compounds. Evidence has been obtained that this series
of ribonucleotide reductase inhibitors exert their inhibitory action
through the scavenging of a tyrosyl free radical intermediate of the
enzyme. On the basis that Didox and its polyhydroxyphenyl congeners
are excellent free radical scavengers and the thesis that the
toxicity but not the antitumor activity of the anthracyclines are
due to generation of a toxic free radical intermediate, Didox was
tested to determine if it could decrease the toxicity to acute and
chronic treatment with the anthracyclines in non-tumor bearing
animals. It was found that Didox decreased toxicity as measured by
morbidity in both acute and chronic treatment regimens employing
daunorubicin in the acute experiment and doxorubicin in the chronic
treatment schedule experiment. These results caused us to
administer Didox in conjunction with doxorubicin in L1210 leukemia
and solid tumor (Lewis lung) bearing animals to determine whether
the combination would be less toxic and more therapeutic.
Synergistic results were seen in both tumor models. The addition of
Didox to anthracycline chemotherapy allows the dosage of the
anthracycline to be reduced and the total antitumor activity to be
increased. For example, at a dose of doxorubicin that only produced
a modest (60%) increase in the life span of the L1210 tumor bearing
animals the addition of Didox to this treatment regimen caused a
marked increase in the average life span and a number of cures (> 60
days survival) was observed. In addition, weight loss and exterior
appearance (unruffled fur) of the dual treated mice was much better
than those animals treated with only doxorubicin.

3   EFFECT OF DIFFERENT SCHEDULES OF CALCIUM ANTAGONIST ADMINI-
STRATION ON THE DOXORUBICIN INDUCED CARDIOTOXICITY IN RAT.

Fabrizio Villani[x], Francesco Piccinini, Elena Monti, Luisa Pa
racchini, Luigia Favalli, Annalinda Rozza, Enrica Lanza, Paola Poggi.
Istituto Tumori, Milano; Istituto di Farmacologia, Università di Milano; Istituto di Farmacologia e Istologia, Università di Pavia (Italy).

Conflicting results are reported regarding the effectiveness of
Ca-antagonists on Doxorubicin (DXR) induced cardiotoxicity. This patho
logy was tentatively referred to calcium overload thus suggesting a
possible role for Ca-antagonists in preventing this adverse effect. Ho
wever, Ca-antagonists were shown to enhance DXR accumulation in tumor
cells while pharmacokinetic data in myocardial tissue are lacking. The
aim of the present investigations was to evaluate the effectiveness of
verapamil (V) and flunarizine (F) in preventing the development of DXR
cardiotoxicity in rat and whether a modification of DXR heart pharmaco
kinetics might be responsible for this effect. DXR was administered i.
v. at the dose of 3 mg/kg x 3 every 3 days for a total of 3 administra
tions. In order to clarify whether V and F prevent the development of
DXR cardiotoxicity by modifying the drug uptake or by affecting delayed effects such as Ca overload, V or F were administered i.p. respecti
vely at the dose of 5 and 10 mg/kg daily according to the following
schedules: A) from day 1 to 21; B) from day 22 to 56. The development
of cardiotoxicity was monitored by measuring predictive ECG parameters
(QaT and SaT duration) and by light and electron microscopy evaluation
of left ventricle excised 7 weeks after the last DXR administration.
Cellular pharmacokinetics of DXR and their modification by V and F were also studied in vitro. Experimental data show that V and F, when ad
ministered according to schedule B, partially prevent the ECG indexes
of DXR cardiotoxicity. V and F do not affect the cellular pharmacokine
tics of DXR in vitro in accordance with the scanty activity displayed
by V and F when administered according to schedule A. Morphological e-
valuation of cardiac damage is in agreement with ECG findings. These
results suggest that the partial protective effect of V and F probably
depends on their prevention of calcium overload while cellular pharmacokinetics of DXR does not seem to play a significant role.

Supported by CNR grants no. 85.02561.44 and 85.02303.44, Special Project Oncology.

4 MECHANISM OF THE REDUCTION OF ANTHRACYCLINE
ANTIBIOTICS AND THEIR IRON COMPLEXES BY ASCORBATE:
RELATIONSHIP WITH THEIR EFFECTS ON LIPID PEROXIDA-

TION. Igor B. Afanas'ev,* Natalia I. Polozova, and
Vladimir I. Gunar. All-Union Vitamin Research Institute,
117246 Nauchny proezd 14A, Moscow, USSR

It is now a traditional point of view that the cardiotoxic action of anthracycline antibiotics is due to the
enhancement of mitochondrial membrane lipid peroxidation
via the generation of oxygen radicals. But it remains
unclear why anthracyclines stimulate NADH-dependent peroxidation and inhibit ascorbate-dependent peroxidation.[1]
To bring a more understanding to this question, we studied
the interaction of ascorbate (AH^-) with adriamycin (Adr)
and aclacinomycin A (Acl) and their iron complexes.

It was found that ascorbate reduced these antibiotics
in both aprotic (acetonitrile) and aqueous media to form
deglycosidation products. When $Fe^{3+}Adr$ was involved in the
reaction, a complicated mixture containing deglycosidation
products was finally obtained. However it was found that
at least in aqueous solution the initial attact of
ascorbate was directed on Fe^{3+} ion and not a quinone
moiety of complex. Thus at pH 5.5 the spectrum of free
adriamycin was obtained immediately after AH^- and $Fe^{3+}Adr$
mixing. As we found that $Fe^{2+}Adr$ was fully dissociated
under these conditions, it was concluded that the
following reaction occurs:

$$AH^- + Fe^{3+}Adr \longrightarrow AH\cdot + Fe^{2+}Adr \rightleftharpoons Fe^{2+} + Adr$$

The ability of ascorbate to reduce $Fe^{3+}Adr$ to Fe^{2+} and
adriamycin contradicts the proposal [1] that the inhibition
of ascorbate-dependent lipid peroxidation by adriamycin is
due to adriamycin chelating iron ions. It is possible that
there are other reasons explaining this effect. For
example anthracyclines may react as scavengers of hydroxyl
radicals generated during the ascorbate-driven Fenton
reaction.

1. E.G.Mimnaugh et al.,Biochem.Pharmacol.,34, 547, 1985.

5 SIGNIFICANT REDUCTION OF DELAYED DOXORUBICIN CARDIOTOXICITY BY ICRF-187 IN RATS. Luigia Favalli[x], Enrica Lanza, Annalinda Rozza, Paola Poggi, Milena Galimberti, Fabrizio Villani, Istituto di Farmacologia e Istologia, Università di Pavia; Istituto Nazionale Tumori, Milano (Italy).

Many efforts have been made in order to identify agents able to reduce antracycline cardiotoxicity. Among the various agents tested ICRF-187 offered the most promising results: it has been examined in different animal models of anthracycline induced cardiac toxicity including rabbit,dog and miniature pig. The present investigations were performed in rats using a model of proved doxorubicin delayed cardiotoxicity. Female Sprague Dawley rats, weghing about 150 g received 3 mg/kg of DXR i.v. weekly for 5 weeks. ICRF-187 was administered i.p. at the dose of 100 mg/kg 30 min before each DXR administration. Cardiotoxicity was monitored by means of electrocardiography (QRS duration, SaT and QaT intervals) and by light and electron microscopy evaluation of left ventricle excised 6 weeks after the last DXR administration. The degree of morphologic lesions was quantitated according to the score system proposed by E. Billingham. Immediately after the sacrifice blood samples were also collected for chemical and ematologic determination. Doxorubicin produced a lack of increase in body weight and a significant loss of weight in both atria and ventricles. ECGs from DXR treated animals showed an irreversible and time dependent prolongation of SaT and QaT in comparison to controls (SaT: DXR 30.2 msec vs. 13 msec $p < 0.05$; QaT: 46.5 msec vs. 26.9 $p < 0.05$). Moreover DXR produced typical morphologic alterations including myocites vacuolization, myofibrillar loss and mithocondria swelling, with a mean morphologic score 0.72 (0.02 in controls, $p < 0.05$). No consistent changes were found in serum Ca,K,Na, and Fe levels, white and red blood cells count and Hb concentration. Pretreatment with ICRF-187 caused a significant reduction of loss in body weight and a slight effect on atria and ventricle weight loss. The drug partially prevent SaT and QaT prolongation in ECG (20.5 msec and 35.2 msec respectively, $p < 0.05$ vs. DXR group). Morphologic changes were significantly lower (mean score 0.12, $p < 0.05$ vs. DXR group). In conclusion these data demonstrate that ICRF-187 also in rats provides a significant protection against DXR cardiotoxicity.

Supported by CNR grant no. 84.02561.44.

6

Characterization of the Cardioprotective Effect of (S)(+)-4,4'-propylene-2,6-piperazinedione (ICRF-187) on Anthracycline Cardiotoxicity. Joyce A. Filppi,* Anthony R. Imondi and Richard L. Wolgemuth. Adria Laboratories, Columbus, OH 43216

(S)(+)-4,4'propylene-2,6-piperazinedone, hereafter ADR-529, (ICRF-187), has been shown to effectively reduce the development of Adriamycin induced cardiomyopathy in animal models. In the present study, the effect of ADR-529 on the chronic cardiotoxicity produced by the Adriamycin analogs, epirubicin and idarubicin was examined. The effect of varying the dose level and time of administration of ADR-529 relative to Adriamycin was also evaluated.

Groups of ICR Swiss mice were injected iv with either Adriamycin (4 mg/kg/inj), epirubicin (5 mg/kg/inj) or idarubicin (1 mg/kg/inj). ADR-529 was concomitantly administered in the contralateral tail vein. The treatment schedule consisted of twice a week injections during the first 2 weeks of the 11 week study. The animals were not treated during weeks 3 and 4. During weeks 5-7 the animals received 6 additional biweekly injections and were sacrificed at week 11. Plastic sections of the hearts were examined for characteristic anthracycline induced damage in a blinded fashion.

Administration of ADR-529 at dose ratios of ADR-529:Adriamycin ranging between 4:1 and 20:1 significantly ($p < .001$) decreased the severity of histological lesions relative to those observed in hearts from animals given Adriamycin alone. Time of administration also was found to influence the amount of protection afforded by ADR-529. A reduction of cardiac damage was observed when ADR-529 was given as early as 2 hours prior to Adriamycin and as late as 2 hours after the anthracycline, however, optimal protection occurred when the compound was given from 30 minutes before to 15 minutes after Adriamycin.

ADR-529 in combination with epirubicin or idarubicin at ratios of 12:1 and 20:1 also decreased the cardiac damage relative to that caused by either anthracycline alone.

These studies demonstrate that the cardioprotective effect of ADR-529 is dependent on the dose and time of administration relative to Adriamycin. They also show that the compound is effective in ameliorating the cardiotoxicity induced by epirubicin and idarubicin.

7 **IMMOBILIZED ADRIAMYCIN: TOXIC POTENTIAL IN VIVO AND IN VITRO.** M.P.Hacker, J.S. Lazo, C.A.Pritsos and T.R.Tritton. Dept. of Pharm., Univ. of Vermont, Burlington, VT 05405, Dept. of Pharm., Yale Univ., New Haven, CT 06510 and Dept. of Biochem., Univ. of Nevada, Reno, NV 89557.

Adriamycin covalently attached to agarose polymers has been previously shown to be actively cytotoxic against several cell types in culture. In this form the drug does not gain access to the cell interior and thus elicits its cytotoxicity via cell surface interactions. A therapeutic application of this finding would be to use immobilized drug as an intracavitary agent. Here we report a nearly complete lack of toxic side effects of immobilized adriamycin given intraperitoneally. Using C57Bl/6N mice we injected i.p. up to 200 mg/kg (containing 4 mg/kg adriamycin) in up to 2 ml volume and followed the progress of the animals for 60 days. This dose of free adriamycin causes ≈40% weight loss but is without effect when administered while attached to agarose. Also in contrast to free adriamycin, the polymer bound drug causes no peritoneal adhesions or inflammation. Microscopic evaluation of bowel, ovaries, peritoneal wall, liver and heart showed no abnormalities. There is a slight thickening of the splenic capsule, but no damage to the organ itself. When tested in vitro in the fetal mouse heart system, we find no evidence of cardiotoxic potential. However, respiratory chain particles do show an inhibition of electron flow in both the NADH dehydrogenase and succinate dehydrogenase pathways, suggesting that the lack of cardiotoxicity may not be an intrinsic property of the immobilized drug, but a consequence of the inability of the polymer to penetrate cells. Overall the results provide a strong impetus to continue the evaluation of polymer immobilization in adriamycin therapy.

8 DEPLETION OF POLYAMINES BY DIFLUOROMETHYLORNITHINE (DFMO) DOES NOT ALTER DOXORUBICIN (DOX) TOXICITY

M.P.Hacker and P.J.Kimberly, Vermont Regional Cancer Center and Department of Pharmacology, University of Vermont, Burlington, VT 05405

The polyamines putrescine (PUT), spermidine (SPD), and spermine (SPM) are simple polycationic molecules thought to be involved in a variety of cellular processes. The interactions of the polyamines with DNA have been the focus of research in a number of laboratories. With the development of specific inhibitors of polyamine biosynthesis, such as DFMO which inhibits the enzyme ornithine decarboxylase, several investigators have reported that modulation of cellular polyamine levels can significantly alter the cytotoxicity of a variety of anticancer drugs. Recently it was shown that pretreating human carcinomas with 5mM DFMO for 48 hr significantly diminished the oncolytic activity of DOX. Since a major dose-limiting toxicity of DOX is cardiotoxicity, it is important to determine the effect of polyamine depletion on DOX induced cardiotoxicity. Using the fetal mouse heart organ culture system (FMH) we evaluated the effect of DFMO on DOX toxicity. DOX caused a dose and time dependent decrease in lactic acid dehydrogenase activity (LDH) and total protein and was used therefore as an index of myocardial damage. FMH exposed to 18 or 180 uM DOX for 48 hr had a 50% or 75% decrease in specific LDH activity, respectively. In contrast, no toxic effects were observed in FMH exposed to 5mM DFMO for up to 96 hr. Polyamine levels in the FMH were determined by fluorescent spectroscopy of dansylated polyamines separated by HPLC. Using this analytical technique, we found that DFMO did significantly decrease the levels of PUT and SPD within 48 hr of exposure. Pretreating FMH with 5mM DFMO for 48 hr followed by 48 hr exposure of DOX and DFMO did not enhance the cardiotoxicity of DOX. These studies indicate that: 1) FMH actively synthesize polyamines; 2) DFMO can inhibit the synthesis of polyamines by the FMH; 3) DFMO is not toxic to the FMH; and 4) depletion of myocardial polyamines does not alter the cardiac toxicity of DOX. These studies lend further evidence supporting the hypothesis that DOX antitumor activity and DOX cardiotoxicity occur through separate mechanisms. Studies supported in part by a grant GM 31091 from the NIH.

9   FUNDAMENTAL STUDY OF BLEOMYCIN-INDUCED PULMONARY TOXICITY IN
MICE. Hisao Ekimoto[*], Kimihiko Takada, Mineaki Okada, Junpei
Ito, Katsutoshi Takahashi, Akira Matsuda, Tomohisa Takita[1] and Hamao
Umezawa[1]. Research Laboratory, Pharmaceutical Division, Nippon Kayaku
Co., Ltd. Shimo 3-31-12, Kita-Ku, Tokyo 115, Japan. [1]Institute of
Microbial Chemistry. Kamiosaki 3-14-23, Shinagawa-Ku, Tokyo 141,Japan.

In order to understand pathogenesis of bleomycin(BLM)-induced
pulmonary toxicity and to find antidotes towards the toxicity, we have
done a series of studies on the toxicity in mice.

BLM was i.v. administered into various strains of mice once daily
for 7 days, and the toxicity was microscopically examined at one week
intervals. Grade of the toxicity observed 5 weeks after the injection
was highest in ICR, C57BL/10 and C3H/He mice, moderate in C57BL/6,
B10·D2, DBA/2, A/J, B6C3F[1] and BDF[1] mice, and lowest in B10·A, B10.BR,
CBA/JN, BALB/c, CDF[1] and CBF[1] mice. Microscopic examinations revealed
that edematous reaction occurred around 1 week after the injection
prior to progressive pulmonary fibrosis. The edematous lesions of the
high responders were severer than those of the low responders except
that BALB/c mice, one of low responders, had severe lesions.

The edematous reaction was thought to be due to oxygen toxicity from
the following results: 1) Grade of the edema in the above strains of
mice was inversely correlated with amounts of tocopherol and ascorbic
acid in the lung except in BALB/c and its F[1] mice. 2) BLM-Fe(II)
caused lipid-peroxidation in vitro and in vivo. 3) Exposure of high
concentrations of oxygen during BLM treatments enhanced the toxicity,
but the pre-exposure to the oxygen suppressed the toxicity.

4) Combination of reducing agents such as ascorbic acid, glutathione
and tocopherol with BLM reduced the toxicity. 5) The combination of
selenite plus glutathione markedly reduced the toxicity.

The progressive pulmonary fibrosis seemed to be associated with
immunological reactions from the following results: 1) Carrageenan,
an anti-macrophage agent, reduced the toxicity. 2) Grade of the
toxicity in ICR nude mice was low, but the toxicity was enhanced by
transfusion of thymocytes of ICR mice. 3) Prednisolone and cyclophosphamide which have immunosuppressive activity reduced the toxicity.

Recently, we observed platelet-including microthrombus before
the occurrence of the edematous reaction. Anti-platelet-aggregating
agents such as ticlopidine, dipyridamole and PGI[2] reduced the edema
and the fibrosis. Impairment of microcirculation systems by the
microthrombus may generate oxygen-derived free radicals to injure
the lung.

10   MURINE STRAIN DIFFERENCES IN LUNG PROCOLLAGEN AND FIBRONECTIN
mRNA AFTER CONSTANT SC INFUSION OF BLEOMYCIN. Dale G. Hoyt*
and John S. Lazo. Dept. of Pharmacology, Yale University, New Haven,
Connecticut, 06510, USA

Murine strains differ in their sensitivity to pulmonary fibrosis induced by bleomycin (BLM): BALB/c mice (B) are resistant
whereas C57Bl/6 (C) are sensitive. The role of altered gene
expression in BLM-induced lung injury was explored in these mice
by determining the time course of changes in mRNAs coding for
extracellular matrix proteins after BLM treatment. Osmotic
minipumps that delivered 100 mg/kg BLM over 7d were implanted
sc in mice. Lung mRNAs for α_1I and α_1III procollagen and fibronectin (Fn) isolated 2, 3 and 4 weeks after implantation were
measured by hybridizing ^{32}P-labeled DNA probes to total RNA
applied to nitrocellulose. Lung weight and total lung RNA were
increased earlier and to a greater extent in C. However, the
content of RNA per gram of lung was similar in both strains.
Total lung α_2I mRNA was elevated 2.4 fold at 3 weeks in C and
not increased in B. Total lung α_1III mRNA increased 4.3 fold
in C at 3 weeks. In B, α_1III mRNA decreased to 0.3 of control
at 2 weeks, and then gradually increased to twice the control
value by 4 weeks. Fn mRNA increased earlier and to a greater
degree in the sensitive C mice compared to B mice: 7.8-fold
at 2 weeks and 12.4-fold at 3 weeks in C compared to 3-fold
in B mice at 3 and 4 weeks. The results indicate that fibrosis
is quantitatively associated with specific increases in procollagen and fibronectin mRNA in mice treated with BLM subcutaneously.

11 AMBROXOL AND BLEOMYCIN(BLM)INDUCED PULMONARY TOXICITY:EXPERI-
MENTAL AND CLINICAL ASPECTS.Maurizio Luisetti*,Ernesto Pozzi,
Mario Salmona and Fabrizio Villani.Istituto di Tisiologia,Università
di Pavia;Istituto"M.Negri",Milano;Istituto Nazionale Tumori,Milano,I-
TALY

The pathogenesis of BLM induced lung toxicity is not yet completely clarified:recent reports suggest the possible role of the derange-
ment of surfactant synthesis by type II pneumocytes.The aim of the p-
resent investigation was to evaluate the efficacy of ambroxol(AMB),an
agent found able to influence the secretory activity of these cells
in some experimental models of drug induced lung injuries,to prevent
the pulmonary toxicity of BLM.Experiments conducted in rats demonstrated that in BLM treated animals(1.5 U intratracheally)an increase of
afflux of inflammatory cells(particulary of neutrophils)accours;in t-
he mean time an early increase of alveolar total proteins and a delayed increase of alveolar phospholipids were also observed.In the AMB
protected animals(4 mg/Kg b.w./day per os)a significant decrease of
the afflux of neutrophils in the alveoli and a reduction of phosphol-
ipid hyperproduction were evident.Morphological evaluation of lung c-
hanges showed a delay of fibrosis appearance in AMB protected animal-
s.Experiments with AMB(90 mg daily per os)were also conducted in a d-
ouble blind versus placebo trial in 25 patients suffering from non s-
eminomatous testicular cancer and submitted to a 3 regimens chemotherapy including BLM,Cisplatinum and Vinblastine or VP 16.Pulmonary function was evaluated before,at the end and 4-6 months after the completion of chemotherapy by means of spirographic parameters and by measuring the single breath CO transfer factor and its components,pulm-
onary capillary blood volume,and diffusing capacity of the alveolar-
capillary membrane.In BLM treated patients an impairment of lung function in the follow up period was observed,which was not significantly prevented by AMB.In conclusion experimental data,which evidenced a
correlation between phospholipids kinetics and fibrosis development,
stress the possible role of alveolar surfactant in the pathogenesis
of BLM lung toxicity.The discrepancy with clinical results remains to
be clarified.
Supported by grants no.85.02191.44 and no.84.02280.56 of the Italian
National Research Council.

12 THE PULMONARY TOXICITY OF BLEOMYCIN IN COMBINATION WITH OTHER ANTICANCER AGENTS IN MICE. John E. Schurig*, Audrey R. Farwell and William T. Bradner. Bristol-Myers Company Pharmaceutical Research and Development Division, P.O. Box 5100, Wallingford, CT 06492 and P.O.Box 4755, Syracuse, NY 13221.

The combination of bleomycin plus Platinol has been shown to increase the pulmonary toxicity of bleomycin in mice (Bradner, et al, this meeting). Other drugs used clinically in combination with bleomycin are mitomycin C and vincristine. In humans, mitomycin C has been reported to cause a low incidence of pulmonary and renal toxicity whereas vincristine is not toxic to these organs. Each of these agents was administered to mice at maximum tolerated doses alone and in combination with bleomycin. Pulmonary toxicity was assessed by measuring changes in lung hydroxyproline content. Neither mitomycin C nor vincristine caused pulmonary toxicity or increased the pulmonary toxicity of bleomycin in these studies. BCNU has been shown to cause both pulmonary and renal toxicity in humans. Treatment of mice with BCNU alone caused increased lung hydroxyproline levels and mice receiving BCNU plus bleomycin had lung hydroxyproline levels that were higher than for either drug alone. However increased blood urea nitrogen levels could not be demonstrated in mice receiving BCNU alone. This suggests that the increased pulmonary toxicity observed with BCNU plus bleomycin was related to direct additive effects of bleomycin and BCNU on the pulmonary tissue rather than enhancement of bleomycin blood levels through the nephrotoxic effects of BCNU.

13 INFLUENCE OF PLATINUM COMPLEXES ON THE PULMONARY TOXICITY OF BLEOMYCIN. William T. Bradner*, John E. Schurig and Abraham Schlein. Pharmaceutical Research and Development Division, Bristol-Myers Company, Syracuse, NY 13221-4755 and Wallingford, CT 06492-7660.

Cisplatin and bleomycin are often used together in a variety of combinations in the treatment of head and neck, testicular, and cervical cancers. Thus there may be concern about enhancement of a particular toxicity associated with these drugs. In the course of studying the pulmonary toxicity of various chemotherapeutics we found that cisplatin appears to be without toxicity to the lungs of normal mice and rats. However, in experiments in which bleomycin and cisplatin were given together, at or near maximum tolerated doses, increased lung damage as measured by tissue hydroxyproline levels was observed in mice receiving the combination of drugs compared to those receiving similar doses of bleomycin alone. Spiroplatin (TNO-6) and carboplatin (JM-8) did not enhance bleomycin toxicity in any experiment. Results with iproplatin (JM-9) were variable. Since it is known that patients with reduced kidney function have more prolonged retention of bleomycin (Crooke, et al., Cancer Treatment Rpts 61:1631-1636, 1977), these results suggest that in those diseases in which carboplatin has comparable efficacy to cisplatin it might be worth investigating the utility of carboplatin in the subset of patients presenting with renal disfunction.

14 ACUTE EFFECT OF CISPLATIN ON TUBULAR FUNCTION IN THE RAT KIDNEY. G. Daugaard*, N-H. Holstein-Rathlou, PP. Leyssac. University Institute of Experimental Medicine, Nørre Alle 73,2100 Copenhagen, Denmark.

The acute effect of cisplatin on proximal tubular function was examined in 9 Spraque-Dawley rats (260-290 g). The lithium clearance method and the transit time-occlusion time method were used for assessing the proximal tubular reabsorption rates of sodium and water. The rats were anaesthetized with halothane. The left kidney was exposed through a midline abdominal incision and the left ureter cannulated. An adjustable clamp was placed around the aorta cranial to the renal arteries for occlusion time (OT) measurements. After collection of a blood sample for lithium and inulin analysis, three serial urine samples were collected. OT was measured immediately after the last urine collection. When urine flow and arterial pressure had returned to the reference levels, transit time (TT) was measured by lissamine green. A new blood sample was collected and infusion of cisplatin 5 mg/kg dissolved in 3 ml of isotonic saline (40 µl/min) was started. The intratubular pressure was measured during the whole study period. At the end of cisplatin infusion urine collections and OT-TT measurements were repeated. The following results were obtained:

	Control	After cisplatin infusion
V µl/min/g KW	7.97+1.64	19.51+4.96*
Cin µl/min/g KW	1387 +112	1210+105
CLi/Cin	0.202+0.029	0.340+0.055*
$e^{-TT/OT}$	0.415+0.016	0.497+0.022*
APRpc µl/min/g KW	771+67	589+45*
APRpr µl/min/g KW	1130+108	829+113*
Δ Pprox mmHg		+1.4+0.2*
CNa µl/min/g KW	7.34+1.95	19.49+5.93*

CLi, Cin and CNa = lithium, inulin and sodium clearance, APRpc and APRpr = absolute proximal reabsorption in pars convoluta (pc) and end of pars recta (pr), Pprox = intratubular pressure, KW = kidney weight, *p<0.05.

The present study shows a prompt and marked decrease in sodium and water reabsorption in the proximal tubules immediately after administration of cisplatin with an increase in intratubular hydrostatic pressure. This data strongly suggests that cisplatin induced nephrotoxicity is initiated by a primary proximal tubular impairment.

15 THE EFFECT OF HIGH-DOSE CISPLATIN ON GLOMERULAR FILTRATION AND TUBULAR REABSORPTION. G. Daugaard*, N. Rossing, U. Abildgaard, N-H. Holstein-Rathlou, M. Rørth, PP. Leyssac. Department of Clinical Physiology, The Finsen Institute, Strandboulevarden 49, 2100 Copenhagen, Denmark.

The effect of cisplatin on glomerular and tubular function was followed in 17 males with germ cell tumors treated with 3 cycles of 40 mg/m² cis-platin and VP-16 200 mg/m² day 1-5 every three weeks and bleomycin 15 mg/m² every week. The cisplatin was mixed in 250 ml of 3% sodium chloride, and the patients were extensively hydrated with 200 ml/hr of isotonic saline during the five days of cisplatin treatment. The lithium clearance method was used for determining proximal tubular reabsorption rates of sodium and water. Glomerular filtration rate measured as 51-Cr-EDTA clearance decreased significantly from 121+8 ml/min to 77+3 ml/min after 3 cycles and remained at this decreased level 3 months after termination of treatment. At the same time, values of lithium clearance were 22+2 ml/min, 26+8 ml/min and 34+7 ml/min. Sodium clearance increased significantly from 0.46+0.09 ml/min to 1.29+0.34 ml/min after 3 cycles and remained significantly increased after 3 months. The absolute proximal reabsorption rate of sodium and water decreased significantly from 13.6+1.0 mmol/l and 99.0+7.9 ml/min to 6.9+1.1 mmol/min and 50.8+8.2 ml/min after 3 cycles, respectively. Three months after termination of treatment these values were still significantly decreased. Urinary excretion of N-acetyl-beta-D-glucosaminidase and beta-2-microglobulin increased significantly during the 5 days of cisplatin infusion in all three cycles, but after termination of treatment the values approached normal levels. An increase in the beta-2-microglobulin/albumin clearance ratio was observed on day 6 in every treatment cycle. On day 9 in every treatment cycle a significant decrease in the same clearance ratio together with a significant increase in IgG/albumin clearance ratio was observed.

In conclusion, these observations suggest, that high-dose cisplatin induces a functional proximal tubular impairment together with a decrease in glomerular filtration rate. This effect can be observed at least until 3 months after termination of treatment. The proteinuria observed during cisplatin infusion is predominantly of tubular origin, while the proteinuria between the treatment periods is mainly of glomerular origin.

16 THE EFFECT OF CISPLATIN ON RENAL HEMODYNAMICS AND TUBULAR REAB-SORPTION IN DOGS. U. Abildgaard*, G. Daugaard, PP. Leyssac, N-H. Holstein Rathlou, O. Amtorp. Department of Cardiology, University Hospital Gentofte, DK-2900 Hellerup, Denmark.

To localize the nephrotoxic action of 5 mg cisplatin per kg body weight i.v., we have taken advantage of the lithium clearance method. Twenty neurolept anaesthetized dogs (17 to 32 kg) were used in three experimental groups: I: In six animals the effect of cisplatin was investigated 0-160 min after administration of the drug. II: In eight animals the effect was investigated 48 to 72 hours after administration of the drug. III: Six neurolept anaesthetized dogs served as controls. The following results were obtained:

	Group I (after 20 min)	Group II	Group III
RBF ml/min	211+14	143+14*	212+8
GFR ml/min	51.0+3.7	10.7+1.1*	49.0+2.0
V ml/min	0.65+0.13*	1.09+0.11*	0.18+0.01
CNa ml/min	0.60+0.23*	0.63+0.10*	0.08+0.02
CLi ml/min	23.76+4.00*	6.29+0.61*	10.15+1.28
APR ml/min	27.22+1.6*	4.4+0.9*	38.8+2.5
ADR Na mmol/min	3.295+0.526*	0.816+0.083*	1.481+0.187

RBF = renal blood flow, GFR = glomerular filtration rate, V = diuresis, CNa and CLi = sodium and lithium clearance, APR = absolute proximal reabsorption rate, ADR Na = absolute distal reabsorption rate of sodium, * indicates $p < 0.05$, group I and II versus group III.

Thus, administration of cisplatin to dogs results in polyuric renal failure. A mainly proximal tubular functional impairment, without alterations in renal hemodynamics are seen shortly after administration of the drug (20 min). 48 to 72 hours after cisplatin the depressed renal function can be attributed to impaired proximal tubular reabsorption rates of sodium and water, associated with increased renal vascular resistance. The polyuria is due to impaired reabsorption rates in more distal nephron segments affecting the concentration mechanism.

17 THE EFFECT OF CISPLATIN UPON PROTEIN THIOL CONCENTRATION IN PROXIMAL TUBULAR CELLS OF THE RAT KIDNEY. Prakash Mistry, Donald J. Spargo*, Patrick A. Riley* and David C.H.McBrien. Biochemistry Department, Brunel University, Uxbridge, UB8 3PH, UK and *Chemical Pathology Department, University College London and Middlesex School of Medicine, London W1P 6DB, UK

The avidity of platinum for sulphur ligands has often been invoked in hypothetical mechanisms explaining the nephrotoxicity of cisplatin. The variation in concentration of low molecular weight thiol compounds such as glutathione in the rat kidney has been reported by several groups. Protein bound thiol groups act as a reservoir of reducing power in equilibrium with the low molecular weight thiols. We have used a cytochemical technique in slices of rat kidney in conjunction with a scanning microdensitometer to measure the concentration of high molecular weight thiol groups in proximal tubular cells at various times after the administration of a nephrotoxic dose of cisplatin (5mg/kg i.p.). Kidneys removed from anaesthetised animals were rapidly cut into 3mm slices, frozen in n-hexane at -70°C and sectioned (5μm) using a cryostat. Sections were air dried, fixed with ethanol and stained for fast reacting thiol groups using DDD and fast blue B (tetraazotised o-dianisidine). The sections were scanned using a computer aided microdensitometer system. Results show that following an initial increase in protein thiol concentration in the proximal tubules 1-3h following cisplatin treatment the concentration drops by 8h and reaches a nadir at 120h post treatment 29% below that of the controls.
The initial increase in protein thiol concentration parallels that reported for glutathione levels. The nadir in protein thiol concentration coincides with the maximal functional disturbance of the kidney as reflected in blood urea levels although the concentration of protein thiols in the treated animals first drops below that of the controls at 8h, long before functional disturbance is manifest.

This work was sponsored by the Cancer Research Campaign.

18 TIME-OF-DAY-DEPENDENT PREVENTION OF CISPLATIN (CP)-INDUCED KIDNEY DAMAGE BY DISULFIRAM (DSF). Reinhard v. Roemeling*, Marie-Christine Mormont, Mark Wick, David Lakatua, Todd Langevin, John Berestka, Jeffrey Rabatin, and William J. M. Hrushesky. Univ. of MN Hospital, Box 414 UMHC, Minneapolis, MN 55455, U.S.A.

CP-induced nephrotoxicity, bone marrow suppression, and gastro-intestinal toxicity are each circadian stage-dependent (Hrushesky, 1984). Many strategies other than drug timing have also been used to decrease CP toxicity. Borch has shown that diethyldithiocarbamate (DDTC) protects mice, rats, and dogs from CP toxicity without interference with anticancer activity. DSF is a DDTC dimer that is rapidly absorbed, reduced to DDTC, and excreted into the urine. It may protect kidney tubule enzymes from irreversible damage. We have tested the rescue effects of DSF in rats following single i.p. injection of CP at one of two times of day, either during sleep (least drug tolerance) or during activity (best tolerance). Rats were randomized to receive DSF or normal saline p.o. concurrently with CP.

Study 1: 50 female Sprague Dawley rats were treated with 11 mg/kg CP with or without 250 mg/kg DSF and were followed for survival. DSF conferred significant survival advantage over saline controls for both treatment timepoints (w = 3.28, $p < 0.02$, two-tailed). Animals treated during activity lived longer.

Study 2: 48 Fischer rats received 11 mg/kg CP and were sacrificed 96 hours later. Quantitative histological evaluation of the kidneys by light microscopy showed less pathological damage in all DSF treated animals ($p < 0.05$). However, only those animals treated at rest had correspondingly lower BUN levels ($p < 0.03$).

Study 3: 50 Fischer rats received 8 mg/kg CP with or without DSF at two dose levels of 250 or 500 mg/kg and were sacrificed 120 hours later. All animals treated with DSF showed somewhat less histological kidney damage (not significant) without obvious dose/effect relationship. Histological damage was slightly less following treatment during activity ($p = 0.09$). Serial determinations of both BUN and serum creatinine levels 48, 96, and 120 hrs after treatment showed a beneficial effect only of high dose DSF for treatment given at rest ($p < 0.05$).

Study 4: 26 Fischer rats with transplantable adenocarcinomas were treated at rest with 5 mg/kg CP with or without 250 mg/kg DSF. DSF did not interfere with CP-induced tumor shrinkage, cure rate, and overall animal survival patterns.

We conclude that DSF protects kidneys from CP-induced damage more or less efficiently depending upon the time of day that CP is given. No interference with CP antitumor activity was observed.

19 AN IN VITRO MODEL FOR INVESTIGATING DIETHYLDITHIOCARBAMATE (DDTC) REVERSAL OF CISPLATIN (DDP) NEPHROTOXICITY. Thomas Montine* and Richard F. Borch. University of Rochester, Rochester NY 14642.

Our laboratory has demonstrated that administration of DDTC following DDP treatment yields reduction in DDP induced nephrotoxocity. It has been suggested that DDP's nephrotoxicity involves coordination of platinum (Pt) to cellular thiols. Experiments in vitro have shown that DDTC can remove Pt complexed to thiol containing enzymes and glutathione. We have employed the LLC-PK$_1$ cell line as a model for studying the mechanistic basis of DDTC reversal of DDP induced nephrotoxicity. LLC-PK$_1$ is an immortal epithelial cell line derived from porcine kidney. When grown to a monolayer these cells express many functions characteristic of proximal tubule epithelia. Cell viablity was assayed by amount of lactate dehydrogenase activity or total protein remaining on the culture plate twenty four hours after drug treatment. Exposure of a monolayer of cells to 100, 200 or 300 uM DDP for one hour results in a decrease in viable cells to 72%, 58%, and 39% of control, respectively. Loss of viability does not begin until approximately 6 hours after 200 uM DDP exposure. Larger doses (up to 400 uM) show shorter times to onset. A five fold greater concentration of trans-diamminedichloroplatinum (II) is required to produce equivalent toxicity. Exposure of a monolayer to DDP (200 uM, 1 hr) followed by DDTC (1 mM, 1 hr) maintains viability up to 93% of controls. DDTC treatment (1 mM, 1 hr) immediately before, immediately after, or 1 hour after DDP (300 uM, 1 hr) exhibited the same degree of protection in all cases. In contrast, thiosulfate (1 mM, 1 hr) afforded protection only when administered immediately before DDP. We have isolated Pt(DDTC)$_2$ from monolayers exposed to DDP (300 uM, 1 hr) followed by DDTC (1 mM, 1 hr). These data support the use of the LLC-PK$_1$ cell line in the investigation of the mechanistic basis of DDTC reversal of DDP nephrotoxocity.

Supported by grants CA-34620 and CA-11198.

20 REACTIVITY OF PLATINUM COMPLEXES WITH SULFUR-CONTAINING NUC-
LEOPHILES. Peter C. Dedon* and Richard F. Borch. Dept. of Pharmacology and Cancer Center, University of Rochester, Rochester, NY,
14642.

The antitumor activity and toxicity of platinum (Pt) complexes
are governed by nucleophilic substitution reactions with a variety of
molecules in the biologic milieu. Sulfur-containing species affect
the biologic activity of Pt complexes in several ways: the proposed
inhibition of enzymes as part of Pt toxicity; glutathione's (GSH) role
as a modulator of Pt complex activity; and the chemoprotection afforded by diethyldithiocarbamate (DDTC) and thiosulfate (TS). We have
studied the reactions of several Pt antitumor agents with sulfur-containing amino acids, peptides, proteins, and nonbiologic molecules in
vitro.

Since GSH serves as a model for protein sulfhydryl groups, experiments were undertaken to characterize the products formed when GSH
reacts with Pt complexes. Under conditions of high Pt concentration
(2-3mM), ^{1}H-NMR and ultrafiltration studies revealed that GSH formed
large molecular weight species with carboplatin (CBDCA) and cisplatin
(DDP) but not trans-diamminedichloroplatinum(II) (trans-DDP). The
complex $[Pt(GSH)_2 \cdot 3 \cdot H_2O]_n$ was isolated from the reaction of 3mM DDP and
6mM GSH and was shown to contain Pt bound to the cys sulfhydryl group.
GSH may modulate the activity of Pt complexes in vivo. GSH (5mM) was
shown to decrease the rate constant of binding of DDP to DNA from
$7.4 \times 10^{-5} s^{-1}$ to $1.7 \times 10^{-5} s^{-1}$ in vitro.

Utilizing HPLC, second-order rate constants were determined for
the reactions of cys, met, GSH, DDTC, and TS with trans-DDP, CBDCA,
DDP, iproplatin (CHIP), and $[Pt(GSH)_2 \cdot 3 \cdot H_2O]_n$. The rate constant for
the GSH-DDP reaction was found to be $1.32 \times 10^{-2} M^{-1}s^{-1}$ at 37°c. A
ratio of 1:1.5:22:6500 was determined for the reactivity of GSH with
CHIP, CBDCA, DDP and trans-DDP, respectively. The ability of these
Pt complexes to inhibit membrane-bound rat renal enzymes paralleled
their reactivities with the smaller nucleophiles. These findings suggest that CHIP and CBDCA may be less nephrotoxic by virtue of reduced
reactivity in nucleophilic substitution reactions.

DDTC and TS, two agents that reduce Pt-mediated nephrotoxicity,
have similar reactivities with DDP: $6.14 \times 10^{-2} M^{-1}s^{-1}$ and 5.70×10^{-2}
$M^{-1}s^{-1}$, respectively. However, TS was virtually unreactive with the
Pt-S bond in $[Pt(GSH)_2 \cdot 3 \cdot H_2O]_n$ while DDTC readily displaced GSH from
this complex $(k = 4.99 \times 10^{-2} M^{-1}s^{-1})$. Furthermore, TS was less
effective at restoring activity to DDP-inhibited enzymes than DDTC.
These findings, along with biologic observations, suggest that DDTC
and TS possess different mechanisms of chemoprotection.

This work was supported by NIH grants CA34620 and CA11198.

21 A PRELIMINARY CLINICAL STUDY OF REDUCED GLUTATHIONE AS A PROTECTIVE AGENT AGAINST CISPLATIN-INDUCED TOXICITY.

Saro Oriana*, Gian Battista Spatti, Silvia Bohm, Sergio Tognella, Michele Tedeschi, Franco Zunino and Francesco Di Re. Istituto Nazionale per lo Studio e la Cura dei Tumori, 20133 Milano and Boehringer Biochemia Robin, 20126 Milano, Italy.

In the attempt to improve the therapeutic index of cisplatin (CDDP) in the treatment of ovarian carcinoma, we have undertaken the clinical evaluation of reduced glutatione (GSH) as a protective agent against toxicity of this antitumor drug. This tripeptide thiol is known to be a safe compound and has been found to be an effective antidotal agent in experimental models. The aim of this study was to assess the feasibility of combining GSH and CDDP in order to provide an equally effective treatment with reduced toxicity. Seven previously untreated patients (6 with advanced ovarian cancer and 1 with primary unknown adenocarcinoma) received CDDP, 90 mg/m^2 (administered IV over 30 min, with standard IV hydration protocol which consisted of 2500 ml fluids) and cyclophosphamide (CTX), 600 mg/m^2 IV every 3 weeks. GSH (1500 mg/m^2, in 100 ml of normal saline) was administered IV over 15 min prior to each CDDP administration. Diuretics were not used on a routine basis. Patients received a total of 45 courses of chemotherapy (33 courses with GSH protection and 12 courses without GSH). Toxicity was essentially gastrointenstinal. Hematologic toxicity was apparently less severe (with nadir leukocyte count >3000/mm^3) than that observed in patients treated with the same regimen without GSH and never required delay of treatment. These preliminary data indicate that GSH can be safely added to the CDDP+CTX regimen in this dose and schedule, since it is well tolerated and produces no unexpected toxicity. Since no nephrotoxic manifestations were observed (peak serum creatinine level of 1.2 mg/dl), we have reduced the volume of fluids (by around 40%) of the hydration protocol in a series of 8 patients treated with the same regimen including GSH (at present, 30 courses). Again no clinical signs of kidney damage were detected. Taken together, these results suggest that GSH may provide protection against cisplatin nephrotoxicity. The therapeutic efficacy of this drug combination was not impaired by GSH pretreatment, since in the previous series 6 complete (pathologically documented) and 1 partial responses were observed. Since this program is both active and well tolerable, as compared to retrospective series, it deserves further studies.

22 MODULATION OF THE TOXIC EFFECTS OF PLATINUM COMPLEXES BY METALLOTHIONEIN. Susan L. Kelley[1]*, Miles P. Hacker[2], and John S. Lazo[3]. Depts. of Medicine[1] and Pharmacology[3], Yale University School of Medicine, New Haven, Connecticut 06510 U.S.A., and Vermont Regional Cancer Center[2], Burlington, Vermont 05401 U.S.A.

Several cellular factors, including thiol compounds, have been proposed to influence the toxicity of cis-platinum (cDDP). Metallothionein (MT), a protein-thiol with 2 isomeric forms, functions in cellular metal homeostasis. We have studied the role of MT in the modulation of cytotoxicity following exposure to cDDP. Human A-253 carcinoma cells were continuously exposed to increasing levels of cadmium (Cd) for 8 months, to a final [$CdCl_2$] of 80 uM. The resulting cell line, A-253CdR, exhibited 10-20 fold resistance to Cd. Rabbit anti-rat MT I+II antiserum was produced and an ELISA was developed to quantitate the cytosolic MT content with a sensitivity of 200pg MT/ug cellular protein. The A-253CdR cells contained a 3-4 fold increase in cytosolic MT content and were 3-fold cross-resistant to cDDP, compared to the parental A-253 cell line. Conversely, cells selected for resistance to cDDP exhibited cross-resistance to Cd. For example, L1210/cDDP cells, which were 30-50 fold resistant to cDDP, were 19 fold cross-resistant to Cd. L1210/cDDP cells contained 13-fold more MT by ELISA compared to the parental cell line. The L1210/DACH cell line manifested 15-fold resistance to 1,2-diaminocyclohexane-Pt-SO_4 (DACH) with 3-fold cross-resistance to cDDP, and 1.8 fold cross-resistance to Cd, when compared to L1210 parental cells. L1210/DACH cells contained a 3-fold increase in MT content. Thus, the levels of cellular MT can modulate the toxicity of cDDP, but do not affect cellular response to DACH. The clinically important toxicities of cDDP may be influenced by the many therapeutic and environmental factors known to elevate cellular MT.

Supported by USPHS Grants CA-01012, CA-25883, CA-43917 and American Cancer Society Grant CH-316. Susan Kelley is the recipient of a Pharmaceutical Manufacturer's Association Foundation Clinical Pharmacology Fellowship.

23 EFFECTS OF PIGMENTATION ON CISPLATIN-INDUCED OTOTOXICITY.
V.G. Schweitzer, M.D.*, R. Turner, Ph.D., S. Raymer, M.
Abrash, M.D. Department of Otolaryngology--Head and Neck Surgery,
Otologic Research Laboratory, and Pathology, Henry Ford Hospital,
2799 W. Grand Blvd., Detroit, Michigan 48202, U.S.A.

The purpose of this pilot project was to evaluate the effects of
pigmentation on Cisplatin-induced ototoxicity and visceral toxicity
with and without the inhibitory agent, Fosfomycin, a phosphonic acid
antibiotic. Recent studies demonstrate that Fosfomycin has a significant protective effect against platinum-induced ototoxicity and
nephrotoxicity when co-administered with Cisplatin at a known therapeutic and tumoricidal dose for Platinol in the guinea pig. The role
of melanin on the susceptibility of albino and pigmented guinea pigs
to ototoxic Cisplatin agents has not been well defined, although,
platinum-induced cochlear toxicity has been demonstrated in both
albino and pigmented animals.

With the guinea pig as a model, the role of pigmentation in platinum induced ototoxicity, nephrotoxicity, and gastrointestinal entero-
pathy was histologically and functionally evaluated by brainstem
evoked auditory response (BSER), cytocochleography and light microscopy of organ of Corti, and light microscopy of kidney and gastrointestinal tissues. Furthermore, gamma emission analysis of ^{195M}plat-
inum localization in inner ear tissues and selected viscera was evaluated in the adult albino and pigmented guinea pig in Cisplatin-
treated and combined Cisplatin and Fosfomycin-treated animals. The
following treatment regimens were used: 1)albino and pigmented guinea
pigs, Cisplatin 0.9 mg/kg/qd s.q. for 12 consecutive days and 2)albino
and pigmented guinea pigs, Cisplatin 0.9 mg/kg/qd s.q. + Fosfomycin
(320 mg/kg/qd s.q.) for 12 consecutive days. BSER was performed pretreatment and at time of sacrifice.

Final data demonstrates: 1)in both treatment groups, albino animals demonstrate more significant BSER threshold elevations at 2, 6,
and 15 kHz and more significant total hair cell loss than the pigmented animals. 2) In both treatment groups, Fosfomycin significantly reduces the total hair cell loss as well as BSER threshold shift at 2
and 6 kHz. 3) Platinum concentration increases in inner ear neuro-
epithelial tissues over 24 hours in contrast to urine, plasma, liver,
lung, kidney and intestine. 4) Fosfomycin significantly reduces
Cisplatin-induced nephrotoxicity.

This study suggests that melanin plays a role in platinum-induced
ototoxicity and that Fosfomycin is a potential inhibitory agent for
Cisplatin-induced ototoxicity and nephrotoxicity. (Supported in part
by grants from Bristol-Myers Pharmaceutical Research Division, Henry
Ford Hospital, and the Deafness Research Foundation).

24

MONITORING FOR CISPLATIN-INDUCED VESTIBULAR TOXICITY: PROSPECTIVE USE OF THE VESTIBULAR AUTOROTATION TEST IN CLINICAL TRIALS. Geli-Ann Kitsigianis, Franco M. Muggia, Steven M. Grunberg, Christy A. Russell, John.R. Daniels, Dennis P. O'Leary. USC Department of Otolaryngology and Comprehensive Cancer Center, 1420 San Pablo St., Los Angeles, CA 90033.

The Vestibular Autorotation Test (VAT) is a new method of computerized vestibular testing, which records and analyzes the vestibulo-ocular reflex. This test is being employed prospectively to document changes from baseline, of patients with previously untreated germ cell tumors and non-small cell lung cancer receiving cisplatin containing regimens at moderate to high dose rates (50-60 mg/m2/week). At completion of a cumulative dose 360 mg/m2 of cisplatin, the first patient studied demonstrated significant abnormalities in vestibular function (Figure 1) in the absence of clinical vestibular symptoms. Correlation with other cisplatin toxicities (cochlear toxicity, neurotoxicity) are being evaluted in these patients, with 14 patients so far being entered into the study. In addition to documenting the presence of subclinical vestibular dysfunction and the possible correlation with other toxicities, this portable, computerized test adds a new dimension in the monitoring of cisplatin toxicities and clinical drug development of platinum analogs. Because the procedure may be performed at the bedside with minimum imposition on patients' scheduling, it becomes feasible to prospectively evaluate protectors of specific toxicities of cisplatin which are in current clinical testing (sodium thiosulfate, WR 2721, and diethyldithiocarbamate). This determination would be particularly useful if vestibular toxicity correlated with cochlear and/or neurotoxicities. We have designed trials of cisplatin ± protector which will be ongoing after initial delineation of parameters predictive for cisplatin toxicity.

25 INFLUENCE OF CISPLATIN DOSE AND SCHEDULE ON CHRONIC NEPHROTOXICITY AND HYPOMAGNESEMIA IN GERM CELL PATIENTS IN REMISSION. Chris Coppin, Division of Medical Oncology, University of British Columbia and Cancer Control Agency of B.C., 600 West 10th Avenue, Vancouver, B.C. V5Z 4E6, Canada

Serum creatinine (S.Cr) and serum magnesium (S.Mg) may be used as simple indicators of glomerular and renal tubular function respectively. Since 1979, patients have been followed for acute and chronic changes in S.Cr and S.Mg associated with cisplatin-containing chemotherapy protocols. Treatment consisted of cisplatin 100 mg/sq.m, bleomycin 90 units, and either vinblastine 12 mg/sq.m or etoposide(VP-16) 360 mg/sq.m every 3 weeks x 4-5 cycles (3 cycles if adjuvant, up to 10 cycles for relapsing patients). Cisplatin was administered as a 6-hour infusion with forced mannitol diuresis, and the dose prorated to creatinine clearance if <100 ml/min in an attempt to reduce chronic nephrotoxicity. Acute changes in S.Mg were followed in 93 patients, and chronic changes over one year in 58 patients in remission, median followup 34 months. Magnesium supplements or dietary modification have not been used.

Timecourse of Recovery of Serum Magnesium:

Months Post:	0	1	2	3-5	6-10	11-15	...	>65
Mean S.Mg:	1.35	1.17	1.43	1.54	1.55	1.66	...	1.67 mg%

No significant recovery was seen beyond a year from Rx. Considerable month-to-month variation in S.Mg is seen: average standard deviation beyond 1 year=0.16 mg%. Three patients have chronic S.Mgs of c.1.0 mg%; one developed hypertension after 3 yrs.

Effect of Cumulative Cisplatin Dose on Chronic S.Mg & S.Cr:

Cycles	Pts	av.mg/sq.m	S.Cr	S.Mg mg%
≤3	12	265	1.10	1.65
4	35	374	1.19	1.64
5	8	482	1.17	1.49*
8	1	733	1.5	1.35
10	2	958	1.3	1.07*

Elevated chronic S.Cr was sporadic and not clearly dose-related. No correlation was observed between chronic S.Mg and acute or chronic S.Cr, and only weakly with rate of acute fall of S.Mg on Rx (P=.06).

High Intensity Cisplatin Protocol

A similar analysis has been done for 14 patients treated intensively with weekly Cisplatin (mean 673 mg/sq.m) and VP-16. Acutely, this produced more severe glomerular damage (mean max S.Cr 2.13*) and about the same rate of fall of S.Mg as with q3week Rx (mean min S.Mg 0.95). At median 5 month follow-up post cisplatin, mean S.Cr is 1.60*, but S.Mg has recovered unexpectedly well (mean 1.87*) though may possibly be supported by reduced filtration. *P<.05

26 LOCALISATION OF PLATINUM COMPOUNDS IN THE MOUSE KIDNEY AND PROLIFERATIVE RESPONSES FOLLOWING INDUCED TUBULAR NECROSIS.

C. Ewen[*] & J.H. Hendry. Department of Radiobiology, Paterson Institute for Cancer Research, Christie Hospital & Holt Radium Institute, Manchester M20 9BX, U.K.

The distribution of Pt-195m labelled cisplatin in the kidney was measured autoradiographically, and compared with that of iproplatin and paraplatin. The dose of cisplatin (15 mg/kg i.v.) was the LD_{50}, and amounts of the other compounds corresponding to equimolar amounts of platinum were used. Cisplatin was distributed and cleared from the kidney approximately at random, but with the other compounds there was a more rapid clearance from the outer medullary stripe. This effect may be responsible in part for the lesser renal toxicity of these second generation analogues, if as suggested by others the pars recta is the main target-cell region for toxicity effects.

Following cisplatin, the labelling index (LI) increased from the control level of 0.2-0.5% to $1.9^{\pm}0.3\%$ at day 14, and then it declined to control levels by day 35-40. No changes were noted after LD_{50} doses of iproplatin (50 mg/kg i.v.) or paraplatin (150 mg/kg i.v.).

Uranyl nitrate (16 mg/kg i.v.) was used to induce tubular necrosis. This agent causes considerable acute cell death, followed by a large increase in LI to 10-15% at day 3-4, returning to control levels by day 7. Treatment with cisplatin 14 days previously, inhibited the response to uranyl nitrate, and the LI reached only 4-5%. No effect of prior treatment with iproplatin or paraplatin was observed. The reduced proliferative response to uranyl nitrate is compatible with clinical reports of lower renal tolerance to secondary nephrotoxic treatment following cisplatin. The reduction could be due to either genetic injury induced in the majority of the tubule cells by the cisplatin, so reducing division capacity, or a selective toxicity of cisplatin for a subpopulation of cells otherwise capable of many divisions. This population may be located in the pars recta.

27

N-ISOPROPYL-P [^{123}I]IODOAMPHETAMINE (IMP). A MARKER FOR
RADIATION INDUCED PULMONARY DAMAGE. N. van Zandwijk*, A.
Zwijnenburg, C.A. Hoefnagel, H.R. Marcuse, J. Lebesque,
H.M. Jansen. Divisions of Nuclear, Internal Medicine and
Radiotherapy. Netherlands Cancer Institute. Dept.
Pulmonary Diseases, Academic Medical Center (AMC),
Amsterdam, The Netherlands.

Recently a new radiopharmacentical N-isopropyl-p-
[^{123}I]iodoamphetamine (IMP), originally designed for brain
scintigraphy has been shown to produce excellent camera
images of the lung, presumably by binding to an
endothelial receptor. We studied pulmonary IMP uptake in
11 patients, who received radiotherapy on the thorax for
lung cancer (5), breast cancer (4) and Hodgkin's disease
(2). IMP scans were compared with those obtained with
microspheres, labelled with technetium-99m, that
consistently showed a similar pattern of disturbed uptake,
indicating that IMP has the characteristics of a perfusion
tracer.
Sequential studies in 5 patients showed that reduced IMP
uptake was encountered in irradiated parts of the lung
still exhibiting normal radiographical appearance. We
therefore believe that IMP is an useful marker for
assessing the extent of one of the earliest events in the
process of pulmonary damage induced by irradiation.

28 ORGAN TOXICITIES IN ANTICANCER DRUG SELECTION AND DEVELOPMENT; A NEW APPROACH. Thomas C. Hall, M.D.*, University of Hawaii Cancer Research Center, 1236 Lauhala St., Honolulu, Hawaii 96813.

Drugs which have selective toxicity to normal tissues, including fetal/embryonic tissues, may have selective toxicity to the specific cancers which arise from such normal tissues. "Histotoxicity" observed clinically has been used in the selection of a number of effective anticancer drugs. Usually there is a narrow range of anticancer effectiveness which parallels clinical tissue toxicity. Often the drug effects are more histotoxic than organotoxic; eg op' DDD effects only the cortex of the adrenal; cisplatin affects the renal tubules selectively, corticoids lyse lymphocytes and not granulocytes. The number of effective anticancer drugs chosen because they were initially observed to be histotoxic to normal tissues is impressive and includes: nitrogen mustard, corticoids, op'DDD, vinca alkaloids, streptozotocin and aminoglutethimide. Current histotoxic agents under clinical trial development include: sangivamycin for gall bladder cancer and pyrazole for follicular thyroid cancer.

Material will be presented on several dozen other compounds which should be considered for drug development based upon selective normal tissue histotoxicity to - fibroblasts, mouth muscle, mesothelium, melanocytes, chondrocytes, osteoblasts striated muscle, kidney, pancreas, pituitary, lung, liver, adrenal, capillaries, seminiferous tubules, esophagus, salivary glands, neurones, bladder, T lymphocytes and duodenum. If this new method of selection for drug development is a fraction as successful as mouse screening, it deserves a try. Details of histotoxicities will be presented.

29 ORGAN TOXICITIES AND ANTITUMOR RESPONSES; ARE THEY PHARMACOGENETICALLY RELATED? Thomas C. Hall, M.D.*, University of Hawaii Cancer Research Center, 1236 Lauhala St. Honolulu, Hawaii 96813

Clinical toxicity to normal organs is of two types: the first is dose related, variable in degree and statistically inferrable from clinical trials. There are some positive relations between drug dose, toxicity and reponses, since clinical cancer chemotherapy operates close to the maximum intended clinical doses. In addition, responding patients tend to be treated beyond the initial "trial guarantee" period and until relapse, with a greater opportunity for cumulative toxicity. A second type of toxicity may also occur: uncommon, sudden, unexpected, not dose or treatment-time related but severe and unexplained except as an idiosyncratic or pharmacogenetic event.

In the latter toxicity, one assumes that certain normal cells or tissues of the host are uniquely drug sensitive; often severe thrombocytopenia, granaeocytopenia and mucositis will occur together, suggesting a generalized genetic sensitivity. Does such extra sensitivity extend to tumors which share the same genetic complement? If so, do tumors arising from intoxicatable tissues, i.e. colon cancers in patients with unexpected severe drug-associated colitis, respond unusually well to the intoxicating agent?

We have examined this phenomenon in protocols of the GI Tumor Study Group and found evidence which leads us to conclude that (1)After a minimally toxic dose is achieved, responses do not increase with toxicity among the general study population. (2) However, severe, uncommon, unexpected and non-dose related toxicity appears to increase the likelihood of tumor response in the same patient to the intoxicating agent. Examples and discussion will be provided.

AUTHOR INDEX

SUBJECT INDEX